Foods Can Save Your Life

Leading Experts Tell You Why

By Neal D. Barnard, M.D.

Published in the United States by
The Magni Group, Inc,
P.O. Box 849
McKinney, TX 75070

Notice to Readers

This book provides detailed information on how food choices improve health. It does not take the place of individualized medical care. If you have any medical condition, are taking medication, or are over forty, please see your doctor before changing your diet or increasing your physical activity. Changes in diet and exercise sometimes necessitate a change in medications or in other aspects of medical care.

Neal D. Barnard, M.D.

Also by Dr. Barnard:
Food Is A Wonder Medicine, The Magni Group Inc., 1996
Foods That Cause You To Lose Weight, The Magni Group Inc., 1992
How To Turn Your Favorite Meals Into Negative Calorie Effect Meals, The Magni Group Inc., 1995
Eat Right, Live Longer, Harmony Books, 1995
Foods That Cause You To Lose Weight II, The Magni Group Inc., 1996
Power Snacks, The Magni Group Inc., 1996

Table of Contents

Introduction

Healthy eating is a gold mine. With the right food selections, you can lose weight permanently, without restrictive diets. You can prevent heart attacks and even reverse existing heart disease. Through a combined approach of life-style changes, as much as eighty percent of cancer can be prevented. Millions of cases of what passes for the "flu" actually came into our homes in our groceries. We can prevent those as well. We can use foods to get a good night's sleep without sleeping pills, and can plan a morning meal that will help us feel alert through the day.

We will look at the best and latest information on healthy eating from leading authorities. These experts usually write for other scientists and doctors, rather than for the lay public. But they have found the very best ways to control weight permanently, to lower cholesterol dramatically, to prevent cancer, and to do many other things through simple and straightforward food choices. You should know about it.

Many of the things I discovered in preparing this book surprised me too. As a doctor, I knew about the importance of nutrition, but, like most physicians, I began my career without taking the time to look at the real state of the art in nutrition research. Years ago, when the University Hospital swallowed me along with the other frightened medical students, we had too much on our minds to think about healthy eating. Our neckties were awkwardly knotted under our collars. Our white jackets were baggy and too short. We were terrified of drowning in the long hours of demanding, detailed work. Nutrition, preventive medicine, and health in general never figured in our minds. With junk food stuffed in our pockets and plenty of black coffee and cigarettes, we were determined only to survive.

Near the end of my medical training, however, I found that there is a wealth of information which is well-known to researchers, but is largely unknown to lay readers.

In this book, I have let leaders in research tell of their findings themselves:

> **Oliver Alabaster, M.D.**, the Director of the Institute for Disease Prevention at the George Washington University Medical Center, **John Bailar, M.D., Ph.D.**, former Editor-in-Chief of the Journal of the National Cancer Institute, **Peter Greenwald, M.D.**, Director of Cancer Prevention and Control of the National Cancer Institute, and **Denis Burkitt, M.D.**, the renowned surgeon and pioneering researcher on the value of fiber, tell of

the War on Cancer and the breakthrough dietary approach to cancer prevention.

Heart surgeon **Michael DeBakey, M.D., and William Castelli, M.D.**, of the Framingham Heart Study, tell of the new approaches to cholesterol and heart disease.

Denis Burkitt, M.D., whose expertise covers not only cancer research but research into other common illnesses as well, **John McDougall, M.D.**, a leading author and lecturer on nutrition, and **Monroe Rosenthal, M.D.**, of the Pritikin Program, describe the new approaches to a variety of common illnesses from constipation to varicose veins to osteoporosis and impotence.

Mitchell Cohen, M.D., of the Centers for Disease Control, and **Carol Tucker Foreman**, the former Assistant Secretary of Agriculture, tell of the uninvited guests that lurk in foods.

Richard Wurtman, M.D., of the Massachusetts Institute of Technology, and **C. Keith Conners, Ph.D.**, of Children's Hospital in Washington, D.C., detail the effects of foods on the mental functioning of children and adults.

Paleoanthropologist **Richard E. Leakey** and leading primate expert **Jane Goodall** give fascinating insights into the history of the human diet.

T. Colin Campbell, Ph.D. and **Anthony Sattilaro, M.D.**, show how traditional Asian diets give a fresh perspective on our own.

In engaging interviews, they tell of their unique perspectives on the power of foods. Each of them has broken new ground. They might not agree totally with each other or with me at times, but each offers an essential piece of the puzzle.

Chapter 1

Cholesterol, Food, and Your Heart

Every day, 4,000 Americans have a heart attack. Those who survive often suffer another heart attack later. But this does not have to occur. To a great extent, we can now control the risk of heart attacks. And we can even reverse existing heart disease.

Atherosclerosis is the all-too-common form of heart disease in which plaques of cholesterol and other substances form in the artery walls. Plaques form very much like small tumors. The process is gradual: As fats and cholesterol deposit in the walls of our arteries, the muscle cells which normally wrap around arteries, giving them strength like steel bands in a tire, start to overgrow. The muscle cells begin to multiply out of control. They form what are essentially tumors inside the artery. These are the plaques—cholesterol, fat, muscle cells, and other debris. They look like bumps on the inside wall of the artery.

The coronary arteries bring oxygen to the heart muscle itself. (They are called coronary arteries because they form a ring around the heart, rather like a crown.) As plaques gradually form, the passageway for blood becomes clogged. Less blood flow means less oxygen for the heart muscle. The heart, then, tires easily during exercise or excitement. Chest pain (angina) occurs. When the blood supply is completely blocked, a part of the heart muscle dies. This is a heart attack (myocardial infarction).

A New Cholesterol Goal

Many studies have shown the connection between cholesterol and heart troubles. Beginning in 1949, the population of Framingham, Massachusetts, has been monitored to see what affects the rate of heart problems. Under the direction of William Castelli, M.D., the study is looking at an entire generation and now, its children.[1]

The Framingham study showed how common heart attacks really are. Healthy men and women were rapidly being picked off by heart disease. In the first 14 years of the study, heart attacks hit one out of every eight men who had been in their early forties at the beginning of the study. Heart attacks felled one out of four who were in their late fifties at the beginning of the study. "When our friends saw those rates," Castelli said, "they all said, 'If I were you I'd get out of Framingham.'"

Not that that would help. Lowering the level of cholesterol in your blood stream, on the other hand, can make all the difference in the world. Castelli found that there is a cholesterol level below which heart attacks essentially do not occur. "We think there is a threshold in cholesterol, and that it's 150," says Castelli. "We've never had a heart attack in Framingham in thirty-five years in anyone who had a cholesterol under 150. Three-quarters of the people who live on the face of this earth never have a heart attack. Their cholesterols are all around 150. They live in Asia, Africa, South America, outside the big cities. All they need to do to get this disease today is to make a lot of money and move to Rio or Buenos Aires or Cape Town or Singapore or Hong Kong or, lately, to Tokyo, and they can get this disease."

> *"We've never had a heart attack in Framingham in thirty-five years in anyone who had a cholesterol under 150. Three-quarters of the people who live on the face of this earth never have a heart attack."*
>
> **Dr. William Castelli**

With the move to the big city comes an increase in meat consumption. We need to do just the reverse. If we adopt a healthier diet, we can cut our cholesterol levels and our risk of a heart attack.

A reading of 150 is lower than the level generally quoted by doctors, who often use 200 as the recommended level. The difference is this: In general, the lower one's cholesterol level, the better, until you get to about 150. Below that point, there is no great benefit to a lower cholesterol (although there is no harm in a lower level). It certainly would be a tremendous improvement if the American population had an average cholesterol below 180 or even 200. But even at those levels, some people will still develop heart disease. It is useful to remember 150 as the number below which heart disease is nearly impossible.

High cholesterols do not come from the air. They come from our plates. There are, in fact, several things we put on our plates that affect our cholesterol levels. The first, of course, is cholesterol itself.

Cholesterol is found in all foods that come from animals: meat, poultry, fish, eggs, milk, cheese, yogurt, and every other meat and dairy product.

Animals, including the human animal, manufacture cholesterol in their livers for use as a building block for sex hormones, cell membranes, and digestive secretions. While the body uses cholesterol for these purposes, it makes plenty of cholesterol for all its needs. We do not need to add any more through our foods. When we do, the result is that cholesterol is left where it does not belong— in plaques in our arteries. The more cholesterol we consume, the higher our cholesterol levels go.

Even worse are saturated fats. Saturated fats are cholesterol-makers. They turn on the cholesterol-producing machinery in your liver. Don't get nervous about these chemical terms. *Saturated* simply means that the fat molecule is covered with hydrogen atoms. A molecule of saturated fat is like a bus with every seat filled. There is no room for another hydrogen atom. The hydrogen atoms generally add on in pairs. If several pairs of "seats" are empty, the fat molecule is called *polyunsaturated*. If just one pair of "seats" is empty, the fat molecule is called *monounsaturated*.

An easy way to identify saturated fats is to note that they are usually solid at room temperature. Beef fat, chicken fat, and most other animal fats are largely saturated. Meats often have fat not only on the outer edge, but also marbled throughout the lean. The worst offenders are processed meats: hot dogs, salami, sausage, bologna, etc. Commercial hamburgers are in much the same category. Castelli says, "When you see the Golden Arches, you're probably on the road to the pearly gates." Even "lean" meats and poultry contain significant amounts of saturated fat (in addition to cholesterol itself).

Vegetable oils are very different. They are high in polyunsaturates or monounsaturates and generally do not raise cholesterol levels, at least not very much. Corn oil, peanut oil, safflower oil, olive oil, and other vegetable oils are in this category.

Tropical oils are exceptions; palm oil, palm kernel oil, and coconut oil are high in saturated fat. They should be avoided. To remember them, picture a palm tree with its coconuts. Read the labels on baked goods. You'll often find tropical oils in commercial products, because they resist oxidation and prolong the shelf-life of products.

Vegetable oils can be chemically changed to saturated fats by a process called hydrogenation. Hydrogenated vegetable oils, then, are solid at room temperature, so they can be used in products such as margarine and maintain a longer shelf-life. But in the process, they are turned into a fat that will raise serum cholesterol.

Reversing Heart Disease

If we have advanced atherosclerosis, can we become healthy again? Happily, the answer is "Yes."

For most of us, plaques form gradually over many years. They begin to clog the arteries that carry oxygen to the heart muscle. They form in the arteries to the brain or to other parts of the body. They eventually lead to serious disability, then death. But, according to Castelli, diet can reverse this process.

"I worked in the 1950s for a pathologist in Belgium," Castelli said. "Every time he did an autopsy he would say, 'They're coming back.'

"We'd say, 'What are coming back?'

"He'd say, 'The plaques are coming back.'

"'Where did they go?'

"He'd say, 'I don't know where they went, but they disappeared.'

"'When did they disappear?'

"'1942.'

"Two years after the German occupation, they disappeared from the arteries of Belgians. Before the war they were there on about three-fourths of the people who died. They disappeared from '42 to '50, not just in Belgium, but in Holland, Poland, Norway, and northern France. The Germans went into all these countries. They backed up trucks to the farms and took all the meat and livestock back to Germany with the able-bodied men to take care of them.

"And so, they went on a vegetarian diet, not because they had read Adele Davis or Nathan Pritikin—there just wasn't any meat to eat, and the lesions disappeared. And of course, now they are back. They're there now on three-fourths of the people who die."

We can get rid of the disease. Evidence shows that plaques can gradually dissolve. Atherosclerosis appears to be reversible. "It will go away," Castelli said. "Get your total cholesterol down to 150, and keep it there for five years. I don't care how you do it. Diet would be the best way, but if you have to use drugs you can still do it. You will reverse your lesions."

A number of studies have suggested that even established plaques can be diminished. Dean Ornish, M.D., is the author of *Dr. Dean Ornish's Program for Reversing Heart Disease* (Random House, 1990). Ornish and his colleagues in San Francisco have shown that a program of exercise, elimination of smoking, stress reduction, and a low-fat, vegetarian diet can yield signs of reversal within one year in 82 percent of patients. It happens gradually. But it will generally not happen unless one's life-style is comprehensively changed. The typical American Heart Association diet, composed of poultry, fish, and "lean meats," is too weak to reverse heart disease for most people. A vegetarian diet is much more powerful.

Toward an Optimal Diet

I asked William Castelli if, after all his years of seeing some people develop heart disease and others remain free of it, he could say which food choices are the best. I asked, not about halfway measures, but about a truly optimal diet. "Well, vegetarians have the best diet," Castelli said. "They have the lowest rates of coronary disease of any group in the country."

But most of us were not raised as vegetarians. While we know that meat and dairy products are loaded with fat and devoid of fiber, a shift toward a meatless diet is not automatic. For some, the best way is to add a few vegetarian meals to one's routine and gradually increase the number of meatless entrees over time. For others, it helps to shift in steps—first, abandoning red meat, poultry, and fish, and later, phasing out dairy products. Castelli suggests a gradual approach. "Most families only eat from about 10 or 12 recipes. They tend to eat the same stuff night after night after night. Any time you make one of those recipes a pure vegetarian recipe, you're going to be way ahead of the game in terms of the total health impact.

"We ought to be helping people to find ways to do this. I tell them, go out and buy all the vegetarian cookbooks you can get your hands on. Try the recipes, one after another, and if you don't like it, don't feel bad, just toss it. On to the next. If you did that, you could find 10 recipes that you'd enjoy, and that would be the secret to success."

We can get plenty of protein without eating meat. "You can get good protein from cereals," Castelli said. "But what we do to cereals in this country is a crime. We take whole grain cereals, and we remove the wheat germ. We stick the wheat germ in a jar, and we sell it to you separately. We take out all the bran and shove that in a box and sell that separately. What's left over we fluff up, puff out, flake, spray on chocolate and strawberries and all this kiddy-goo stuff. And that's what we get to eat for breakfast.

"Now they're taking the bran that they took out initially, and they're spraying that back on. So we have all these new fiber-enriched cereals. The problem with some of them is that they spray on coconut oil at the same time. The reason they use coconut oil is that it's a totally saturated fat, and it resists oxidation. So the flakes stay crispier longer. The flake who ate it, however, did not stay crispier longer."

But the good news is finally here. Heart disease can be stopped. And the dietary changes that prevent or reverse heart disease also help prevent cancer, help keep our weight down, and prevent a whole host of other common problems. If we can get over a few hurdles of dietary change, we find ourselves in a whole new race. Our lives will be longer and healthier; our spouses and children—and even our parents—can be active and healthy well into a ripe old age.

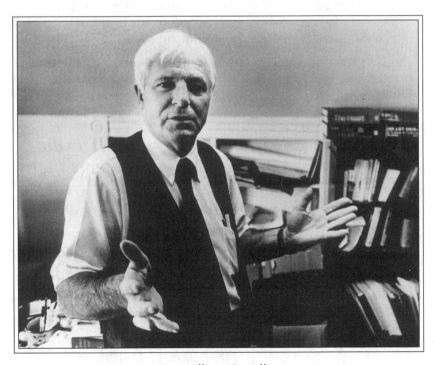

Dr. William Castelli

Chapter 2

Dr. Michael DeBakey: An Interview

Michael DeBakey is a pioneer in heart transplants, bypasses, and the artificial heart, and the author of countless medical publications. Although he has spent decades in the operating room undoing the damage of unhealthful dietary habits, in the past several years DeBakey has often beaten his scalpel into a plowshare, educating patients on healthier ways to eat so as to prevent the need for the operations he has developed. Although he is a demanding and meticulous researcher, he is a warm and friendly man who is generous with his time and his ideas. He fondly recalls the spiced rice and beans of his Louisiana youth, which probably were far lower in fat than most "prudent" heart recipes.

Barnard: Do you feel, as a cardiovascular surgeon over so many years, that you have been working to undo the damage that people's life-styles have been doing to them?

DeBakey: We see so many cardiovascular problems that we have to deal with surgically, and then we see these same people afterwards going back to their old life-styles. You take care of their immediate complaints, and as they begin to feel normal, they slip right back into their old habits. It really is important to educate them.

Barnard: Does that mean that a heart bypass will fail if they don't change their diet?

DeBakey: There's no question in our minds that the risk is greater if they tend to continue with a high-fat diet.

> *"We see so many cadiovascular problems that we have to deal with surgically, and then we see these same people afterwards going back to their old life-styles. It really is important to educate them."*
>
> **Dr. Michael DeBakey**

Barnard: People may feel that changing their diets won't help because there may be hereditary factors in heart disease.

DeBakey: It is true that a small percentage of patients have a hereditary form of arteriosclerosis in the sense that in their immediate family and their parents' and grandparents' families, there is a high incidence of atherosclerosis and coronary disease. Then, there is a form of hyper-cholesterolemia, hyperlipoproteinemia, that is definitely genetic. But that only constitutes about five percent of the cases. So I believe that most people don't really have hereditary disease.

Barnard: Is there a time when a person is too old to benefit from changing the diet?

DeBakey: No, we don't think so. We strongly recommend to people in their sixties and even in their seventies that I operate on, to go on a definite dietary regimen. And if they've been on a high-fat content diet, we strongly urge them to reduce the fat content to maybe 20 to 30 percent.

> *"We strongly recommend to people in their sixties and even in their seventies that I operate on, to go on a definite dietary regimen. And if they've been on a high-fat content diet, we strongly urge them to reduce the fat content to maybe 20 to 30 percent."*
>
> **Dr. Michael DeBakey**

Barnard: Your book, *The Living Heart Diet,* includes international foods, beans and rice, for example, which I suppose most people here don't eat, but in Mexico or other countries are much more common.

DeBakey: Yes. We have them here, and they're good. People in certain parts of the country, like my part of the country, south Louisiana where I was born and reared, eat rice every day. Bean dishes are also popular. Beans were formerly considered poor man's food. We have several menus in the book for beans and rice that are delicious. I've had them myself, and my wife, who is a good cook, has used them and likes them. There are rice recipes in the book that are quite good: brown rice, white rice, enriched rice, with and without salt, and so on.

If rice is prepared properly, it's very tasty. The trouble is most people think of rice the way the Chinese prepare it. They like it that way, but we prepare rice with something else, so that the rice is not just boiled. It can be mixed with herbs to make it very tasty. Rice and beans are good foods.

Barnard: Good for longevity. How have you avoided coronary artery disease in your own life? Are you jogging every morning?

DeBakey: No, I don't jog.

Barnard: I don't get the impression you take many vacations, looking at the list of articles and books you've written.

DeBakey: No, I don't take vacations. I do a lot of travelling, both in the States and overseas. I just returned from Australia. I went to Chicago this past week. Next week I'm going to Costa Rica. In a couple of weeks I have to go to Europe. Because I do so much traveling, I don't take formal vacations. And because I'm active all the time, I don't take formal exercise; I usually try to use the stairs here. I walk up and down these stairs from the operating room, which is six floors down. So that gives me a bit of exercise. I main-tain a pretty active program. And I'm a very moderate eater.

Barnard: In terms of quantity?

DeBakey: Yes. I love vegetables and fruits. I really have only one meal a day, usually in the evening when I go home.

Barnard: No breakfast or lunch usually?

DeBakey: A piece of fruit.

Barnard: A piece of fruit for breakfast.

DeBakey: And lunch may be just yogurt or something like that. Lunch for me is not a specific time because of my operating schedule. I don't know what time I'll be out of the operating room. I may be out at ten or I may not be out until three.

Barnard: How about children? Children love ice cream, they love McDonald's. Should they be taught differently from an early age?

DeBakey: Yes. I think so. We've done that in our family with my children. I have an eight-year old daughter, and she's never eaten anything at a fast-food restaurant.

Barnard: Your daughter has never been to McDonald's?

DeBakey: Well, she has gone to such places with some of her friends, but because my wife and I have strongly urged her not to eat any fast foods, she will go in with her friends maybe for a little bit, but she won't eat anything. She's never had a hamburger from those places because we don't want her eating that kind of food. We want her to learn to like the kind of food that we have on the table.

Barnard: I wonder about this in the hospitals. When I go in the hospital cafeteria, they've got a lot of nice developments, but they're all toward making the food more attractive. They have a dessert bar and so on.

DeBakey: You're quite right about that. I don't know the reason for it. I suppose the cafeteria is a section of some department and they hire cooks and leave it at their discretion, but the cafeteria should be under the control of a good nutritionist.

Barnard: Many hospital nutritionists in my experience are still saying a lot of outdated things—the old "four food groups" and so on.

DeBakey: You're right.

Barnard: Some probably wouldn't like your own dietary habits and would counsel you to have more meat in your diet and so on. I think it's appalling.

DeBakey: Yes, I agree. I don't eat in the cafeteria here, and I don't know what kind of cafeteria we have. I hope it's not that bad. I just got back from Illinois, and although I didn't eat in the cafeteria, we went through to get a cup of coffee, and I saw what they had. You're absolutely correct.

Barnard: How did Americans get on this diet we're on that seems to be so destructive?

DeBakey: I think to some extent it's simply due to the fact that our country's so much better off economically. You don't see this kind of a diet in poor countries where the economic level of the people is low. They eat very little red meat because meat is too expensive. Now the fast-food chains have centered on hamburgers, filled with oil that they're cooked in, with french fries also cooked in oil. It's largely, I think, the economic development of the people in this country that has created that kind of a diet. The Western Europeans are similarly affluent. But the diets of South and Central Americans, Africans, Indians, and Chinese contain little fat and little meat, and they're better off for it.

Barnard: You mention in *The Living Heart Diet* that cholesterol is mainly in the lean portion of meat. Trimming the fat helps, but most of the cholesterol will still be there.

DeBakey: Yes, that's why you have to control the amount. Restaurants serve you a tremendous steak—too much for one person. I don't order steak. If I'm at a banquet or some place where I don't have an opportunity to order, I usually don't eat much of what is served.

Barnard: What's ahead in terms of your own practice and research interests?

DeBakey: Arteriosclerosis/atherosclerosis is my main concern, and the one I'm giving the most attention to. Some of it is clinical in the sense that we're trying to assess what I've done clinically, so I follow my patients. I have records that I'm analyzing all the time. And some is more research-oriented, in perhaps developing ways to deal with certain problems that we have not yet solved, particularly end-stage heart disease. We are trying to find out if there is some way we can open up arteries that are clogged all the way. So we're doing both clinical and experimental work in various areas.

Barnard: How is the work developing for end-stage patients?

DeBakey: I would say for end-stage coronary disease, I suppose cardiac transplantation right now is the best. We're getting about an 85 percent first-year survival rate and projecting a 50 percent five-year survival rate. And it may be closer to 60 percent five-year survival. So, right now that's the only answer we have. The trouble is, of course, that that's limited because you have limitations on the donor. At least 40 to 50 percent of patients that we consider candidates for a transplant die before we can find a donor.

Barnard: How do we deal with the lack of availability of hearts?

DeBakey: Mostly, I think, by trying to educate the public to be more understanding and therefore to give permission. Probably part of the problem is that it's always a tragedy, and the potential donor is relatively young. Young healthy people don't usually die of disease. They die from accidents, and it's always tragic and sudden. The last transplant I did was about five or six days ago. The donor was a 17-year-old boy who shot himself. A tragedy. We had another donor, also a 17-year-old boy who was playing with his friends, and he happened to be sitting on a car that was moving, not rapidly, but he fell off and hit his head some way and had brain death. It's very difficult at that point to talk to the family to get them to give permission. So we have to educate the public, and I think this is being done, but right now we're only reaching about 30 percent of available donors.

Barnard: What do you think of the proposals for animal donors?

DeBakey: It is not feasible right now because we simply don't have a way of controlling the rejection adequately. Cross-species rejection is so severe, and there's not much chance right now of controlling it. It may be possible some day, when we have a

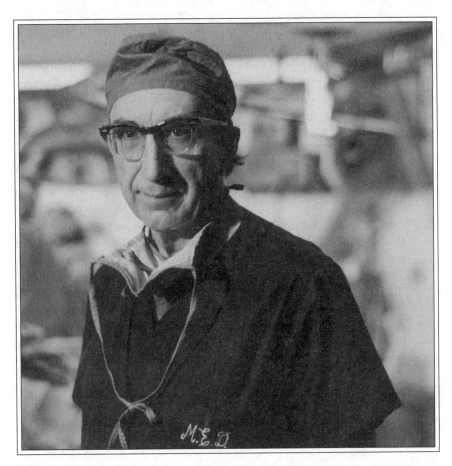

Dr. Michael DeBakey

better understanding of some of the genetics involving the immune mechanism of the body—to modify that without destroying the whole immune function.

Barnard: So when Leonard Bailey put a baboon heart into Baby Fae—

DeBakey: The baby never had a chance.

Barnard: He says it's because he failed to match the blood types.

DeBakey: It wouldn't have made any difference.

Barnard: I guess what was disturbing was that there was the Norwood repair procedure that might have been done for her hypoplastic left heart.

DeBakey: Yes. He obviously was determined to do it. And I questioned him at a symposium on transplants and implants that I was asked to moderate in Louisville. He wasn't on the program. He just appeared and asked for time to present his experience. And I said, "Surely." I questioned him about the incident rather sharply. I asked him to give any evidence that would provide support for doing the procedure. And he said the evidence was his own experimental work. I asked, "What reports have you published?" He replied that they hadn't been published yet. And I said, "Can you give a summary of what you found?" And he did. I said, "Did you have any long-term survivors at all?" His reply was "No."

Barnard: In the animal work?

DeBakey: Yes, he did cross-animal work. Cross-species. Anyway, he said he thought a baby—an infant at that stage—the immune mechanism was not very strong, hadn't been developed well. And he thought with cyclosporine he might be able to hold off until he could find a donor. And I said, "Did you look for a donor first?" He said he didn't. I asked if he planned to do it anyway. And he admitted that he did. I really think that what he did does not have adequate scientific basis. I doubt seriously if you'll see it repeated.

Barnard: I understand this was only the first of a series of five they'd planned to do. Perhaps they're concerned that that might lead to some legal troubles.

DeBakey: I don't know. They've been criticized for it.

Barnard: This brings up the whole question of animals in research. You know, we had a flap about this at the military medical school in Bethesda, Maryland, the Uniformed Services University of the Health Sciences. They were going to shoot dogs to teach debridement, that is, the "cleaning up" of gunshot wounds. I ask you this also because of your wartime experience. The argument the military makes is that a high-velocity wound looks so different from a typical gunshot wound that you have to practice on animals. But I should think debridement principles would apply to all wounds.

DeBakey: No, the trouble is that there is a difference. There's no question about it. We learned that in World War II. The question is whether you need to shoot animals to teach physicians how to debride wounds. I'm not really sure that's necessary. I'm one of the consultants at the Uniformed Services University, and I understand some of their concerns and some of the things they're trying to learn about high-velocity wounds—the extent to which damage is done beyond the surrounding area. Some research is needed in that area. But I think it has to be very specific.

Barnard: I think we, ourselves, have to cut out those uses of animals that are clearly unnecessary. For example, when I was in medical school we didn't learn blood-drawing (venipuncture) on animals. We learned it on the guy in the next desk. I learned to intubate on a patient.

DeBakey: I agree with you. I don't think we would learn that sort of thing on animals in our institution. We teach them how to do these things—venipuncture, intubation, gastric tubes—on humans because we're doing them on humans.

Barnard: Cutdowns, chest tubes, and so on?

DeBakey: Yes. We have to do them on humans to treat them. Why shouldn't the student learn on humans? I gave up surgical training of our students and residents on animals years ago. We used to have a course. I stopped it completely. I said, "I'm not going to do this anymore on animals because we're going to put students in the operating room with humans."

Barnard: How about teaching the techniques of vascular surgery or open heart surgery?

DeBakey: You don't have to have a living animal to try to do microsurgery, say to repair a vessel. You can use fresh cadavers.

It's very easy. You just take a piece of tissue out of a fresh cadaver, whether it's an animal that died from some other reason or a human.

Barnard: Is that how you train the residents here—cadavers?

DeBakey: Yes.

Barnard: And I guess the operating room is a place for a kind of apprenticeship for residents, where they can observe and gradually take over under supervision.

DeBakey: Absolutely. A lot can be done if one thinks.

Barnard: As opposed to—

DeBakey: Well, as opposed to accepting some tradition or previous way of doing things without thinking about it.

Chapter 3

Tackling Cancer

There is a way to beat cancer. It is not found in the newspapers generally. Every press release of a "breakthrough" drowns in the wave of ever-increasing death rates. But there is a new approach. We now know that the vast majority of cancers *can actually be prevented.*

Time For A New Strategy

"CANCER TESTS: FLOOD OF HOPE,
AN EXCITING FIRST STEP"

read the headline of *USA Today*. Eleven patients with advanced cancer had improved. One had had a complete disappearance of the disease. The miracle drug was interleukin 2. The miracle worker was a researcher at the National Cancer Institute. Calls flooded in. Dying patients and their relatives seized on the hope that, at the eleventh hour, long after hopes carefully constructed between doctor and patient had been bitterly relinquished in the onslaught of cancer, at last, the long-awaited cure was here. The doctor looked clean and confident in the accompanying picture. One patient, a father of five, had faced a certain death from advanced skin cancer. But now he felt "hopeful for the future. There are visible signs I'm getting well. I'm excited. My whole family is excited. I don't know why we've been so blessed."

But it was not to be, at least, not yet. He died six months after the *USA Today* article appeared. No patient on the interleukin 2 treatment had been cured. It was not a silver bullet. Barely a year after the media burst, a harsh editorial in the *Journal of the American Medical Association* (*JAMA*) stated "One would . . . hope that investigators will suppress the urge to publicly state or imply that a breakthrough has taken place until solid evidence exists . . ."[1] Interleukin 2 seemed to be little better than other chemotherapies. It was also extraordinarily poisonous. The editorial called the treatment "an awesome experience" with "devastating toxic reactions" and "astronomical costs." The researchers acknowledged that interleukin 2 was "very toxic . . . very cumbersome and very expensive" and that it had contributed to the deaths of four patients.

Interleukin 2 had followed on the heels of alpha-interferon and other anti-cancer drugs which were widely hailed, only to prove disappointing. "We are definitely not winning with respect to treatment," says cancer researcher John Bailar, M.D., Ph.D. Bailar had been a career researcher at the National Cancer Institute (NCI), and for years was Editor in Chief of the *Journal of the National Cancer Institute*. He had slowly and carefully gone through the figures of what the War on Cancer had—and had not—accomplished. We are losing—losing more patients than ever, losing this medical Vietnam, a war in which we lack the vision we need to win.

John Bailar is a large man. Sporting a moustache and shirt sleeves, he appears surprisingly casual for one of the leaders in cancer research. He has the sturdy look of a Teddy Roosevelt with a kind demeanor and professorial patience.

"There have been some very important advances in cancer treatment over the last three decades," Bailar said. "But with respect to the cure of cancer, they are limited largely to the cancers that tend to occur in children and young adults, and those make up only perhaps one or two percent of the total cancer burden."

Unfortunately, we have only managed to impact on the more rare malignancies with little effect on the most common and deadly forms of cancer. There have been some advances in alleviating cancer, but cures for the most common cancers, unfortunately, remain out of reach.

> *"There have been some very important advances in cancer treatment. But with respect to the cure of cancer, they are limited largely to perhaps one or two percent of the total cancer burden."*
>
> **Dr. John Bailar**

"Cancer death rates continue to go up year after year," Bailar said. "Now, these are real increases. I've taken out the effect of the changing size of the population, the changing age structure, declining mortality from other diseases, and we look at what's left. There is a genuine increase in the frequency of deaths from cancer, and this has been going on quite steadily for a number of years now."

Like the bad news given by a doctor to a cancer patient, his message was met with hostility and defensiveness by many with a stake in research for cancer treatments. But further studies have shown precisely the same thing.

Lung cancer is going up because of tobacco; cancer treatments can do little to stem the death toll. Bailar states, "There is a long lead time between the initiation of smoking as a regular habit and the appearance of lung cancer," Bailar said. "It may be twenty, thirty, forty years or more for some people. So, what we're seeing now is the effect of the rise in tobacco use several decades ago. I think that in years to come we'll see the effect of the curtailing of smoking that is going on now. It just takes a long time to do this."

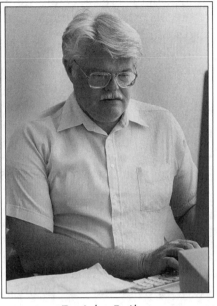

Dr. John Bailar

For breast and prostate cancer, the death rates are not improving. For colorectal cancer, there is a gradual decline, but it is quite slow. Stomach cancer and cervical cancer are occurring *less* often, but when they do occur, treatment is essentially no more effective now than it was decades ago. Year after year, these diseases take a tremendous toll. It is not that researchers are not trying. They simply are not succeeding.

"The degree of improvement in death rates in general for the common cancers of adults is really pretty discouraging," Bailar said. "It has not been for lack of effort. We have poured vast amounts of money into the search for cancer cures over a very long period of time. We've brought some of the best research minds we have to bear on these problems, and it just hasn't worked."

Eighty Percent Preventable

Instead of struggling—and failing—to cure cancer after it has developed, can we prevent it from occurring in the first place? If cancer is caused by environmental or life-style factors, then it potentially can be prevented. In fact, the National Cancer Institute estimates that as much as eighty percent of cancer cases theoretically can be prevented. Some estimates are even higher.

In 1982, the National Research Council released a technical report, *Diet, Nutrition, and Cancer*, showing that diet was probably the greatest single factor in the epidemic of cancer, particularly for cancers of the breast, colon, and prostate.[2] Since then, evidence for effects of certain foods on the incidence of other types of cancer has also steadily accumulated.

Dietary changes are the light at the end of the tunnel for those looking for a way to reduce the cancer epidemic. By avoiding foods that lead to cancer and including foods that strengthen us against the disease, we can, to a great extent, control our own risk.

Fats and Oils

Foods rich in fats and oils increase our cancer risk. Americans certainly eat a lot of fat. About 40 percent of all the calories we eat come from the fat in meats, poultry, fish, dairy products, fried foods, and vegetable oils. Of the many forms of cancer promoted by a high-fat diet, probably the best-studied is breast cancer. A major study by Bruce Armstrong and Richard Doll compared countries with varying diets and found a strong correlation between the per capita consumption of fat and the breast cancer rate.[3]

"Japanese women have the lowest breast cancer rate in the world," said Oliver Alabaster, M.D. "Many Japanese women have migrated to Hawaii and to the U.S. mainland. While marrying within their own community and keeping the population relatively unchanged genetically, they shifted their diet toward a more Western, higher-fat diet, and their breast cancer rate steadily climbed. Within one generation it approximated that of Caucasian women living around them. This is very dramatic evidence that cancer is mainly environmentally induced, rather than genetically inherited." And within Japan, women of high socioeconomic strata who eat meat daily have more than eight times the risk of breast cancer compared to poorer women who rarely consume meat.[4] The most likely culprit is the fat in the meat.

Alabaster is Director of the Institute for Disease Prevention at the George Washington University Medical Center. Alabaster knows about breast cancer; he lost his own mother to the disease. Her cancer was diagnosed at the age of 41. She had a mastectomy and radiation treatments, the standard techniques at the time. But seven years after diagnosis, she succumbed to the advancing illness.

Alabaster was the first to write a simple, convincing guide for the layman on how to prevent cancer. *The Power of Prevention*

(Saville Books, 1986) shows how to take one's risk in hand and actually change it. In reviewing the evidence, he became convinced that fat in the diet was a major contributor to breast cancer, an opinion shared by the National Cancer Institute.

"There is a great deal of evidence that fat increases cancer risk," agrees Peter Greenwald, Director of Cancer Prevention and Control of the National Cancer Institute. "Certainly for breast cancer, when people move from one country to another their risk changes, and the only solid explanation that we have relates to dietary fat. We have a number of case-control epidemiologic studies consistent with this effect. There's a lot of evidence."

The differences in breast cancer rates across various countries are not due to industrialization or air pollution or stress, as Greenwald points out. "There are industrial countries like Japan with low colon and breast cancer rates," he said. "It's not just being industrialized that gives you the high cancer rate. There are rural countries such as New Zealand that have Western habits, and they have the higher cancer rate."

The problem is dietary, particularly the amount of fat we consume. "Fat" in this context refers to all types of fats—animal fats and vegetable oils. Where do we get all this fat? Meats, poultry, fish, whole milk and other dairy products, oily salad dressings, margarine, and fried foods are all sources. Even supposedly "lean meats" contain significant amounts of fat. That goes for chicken and fish as well. The leanest beef is 29 percent fat, as a percentage of calories. Skinless chicken white meat is about 23 percent fat. Fish vary from a low of about 8 percent for cod to well over 50 percent for mackerel, herring, and some types of salmon. Most fish are in the range of 20-30 percent fat. But beans are only four percent fat. Rice is only 1 percent fat. And no plant foods contain any cholesterol. "If you look at the constituents of poultry and fish, they both contain fat," Alabaster said. "It's not as if you're getting on a fat-free diet by eating poultry and fish. They still contain fat, and they contain cholesterol. Fish and poultry are the safest forms of meat, but yet they're still totally different from vegetables, whole grain cereals, fruits, and so on. Breads, cereals, fruits, and vegetables contribute very little fat, a lot of fiber, and no cholesterol. It's only what you then add which is contributing the fat and cholesterol: oils, meats, including fish and poultry for that matter, or dairy products."

How fat in the diet leads to cancer is still poorly understood. Fat is known to affect the activity of sex hormones, which, in turn, may promote certain forms of cancer. Low-fat and vegetarian diets are known to reduce the levels of female sex hormones in the blood stream, particularly estradiol, one of the naturally occurring estrogens which regulate the reproductive cycle.[5,6] Women on high-fat diets tend to have higher levels of these hormones. Sex hormones are known to promote cancer of the breast and the reproductive organs. These observations also suggest a reason behind the young age of puberty in countries where a high-fat diet is consumed. A century or two ago, puberty in girls occurred at about age seventeen. In rural Asian and African countries puberty still occurs in the later teens.[7] But in America and other Westernized societies in the past several decades, the increasing amounts of fat in the diet have been accompanied by the gradual drop in the age of puberty, probably because of abnormal elevations of sex hormones.

Fiber

It is ironic that fiber—the part of the diet which is defined by its indigestibility—should show such power in maintaining our health. But it certainly does. The critical scientific work which established the value of fiber was done by Denis Burkitt, M.D. In his twenty years of surgical practice in Africa, Burkitt wondered why diseases which were so common in England and America were almost never encountered in Africa. The critical factor, he found, was fiber. Fiber passes undigested through the small intestine. It acts to speed the passage of food and to remove harmful substances. The refining processes of developed countries remove the fiber from grains, leading to a high incidence of several diseases. Burkitt found a particularly important connection between fiber and cancer of the colon and rectum.

> *"Of all cancers, colon cancer is the one which is most characteristic of modern Western culture. Colorectal cancer is always rare amongst primitive people. Everything points to diet, and the most important things in diet are fat and fiber."*
>
> **Dr. Dennis Burkitt**

"Of all cancers, colon cancer is the one which is most characteristic of modern Western culture," Burkitt said. "Colorectal cancer is always rare amongst primitive people. It is nonexistent in undomesticated animals. The only animals that get it are highly domesticated animals like dogs and pigs. Everything points to diet, and the most important things in diet are fat and fiber."

Here, again, fat is a culprit. But, to an extent, fiber helps counteract its effects. After a meal, the gallbladder releases bile acids into the intestine to help absorb the fats we have eaten. Bacteria in the intestine turn these bile acids into cancer-promoting substances called secondary bile acids. And this is where fiber comes in, as Dr. Burkitt points out, "Fiber in the diet alters the bacteria in the intestine and reduces the breakdown of primary into secondary bile acids. In addition, fiber absorbs these bile acids the same way that blotting paper absorbs spilled ink. It gets them out of the way. It also dilutes them into a large stool instead of a small stool. So they are reduced, absorbed, and diluted. So in a nutshell, fat would seem to be promotive, and fiber would be protective."

Bile acids are normal. We need them to absorb fat and for other digestive functions. But when these bile acids change into cancer-causing secondary bile acids, we need fiber to minimize this process and to get them out of the way.

Just as colon cancer is rare in countries with a high-fiber diet, a similar pattern is evident with breast cancer. In part, this is because a diet that is high in fiber tends to be low in fat, and a low-fat diet helps reduce risk of breast cancer. But the story is more complex than that. Fiber, it appears, actually offers additional protection.

"There's some evidence suggesting that fiber may be protective against breast cancer," Burkitt said. Again, changes in sex hormones may be responsible. But it is not only dietary fat which changes them; fiber affects hormones as well. "The risk of breast cancer is directly related to the age of menarche, the age when girls reach puberty. In America in the middle of the last century, puberty started at seventeen. Now it's thirteen. In an African village it will be seventeen; in Johannesburg it will be thirteen. A group in Wales under a man called Hughes looked at 46 countries to see what he could find related to age of menarche, and the only thing that related to age of menarche was fiber intake. Fiber affects cholesterol metabolism, and cholesterol is a precursor of the hormones that regulate uterine growth."

By increasing fiber intake, cholesterol levels are reduced. The theory, then, is that reducing cholesterol, in turn, may reduce the levels of hormones which lead to cancer. A second mechanism comes from the fact that waste estrogens are excreted into the intestine via the bile ducts, along with the digestive juices. Fiber helps carry them away. If there is not much fiber in the diet, these waste estrogens can be reabsorbed back into the bloodstream. Of course, increasing fiber intake generally also means decreasing fat intake. In any case, the result is less breast cancer. For now, these are theories, but they help explain the dramatically different ages of sexual maturity and the marked differences in breast cancer rates in groups with different diets.

"Breast cancer is also related to a longer period elapsing between the onset of puberty and the first full-term pregnancy," Burkitt said. "Now if you have a late menarche, then you don't have a long time between menarche and first pregnancy." And your cancer risk is reduced.

If a low-fat, high-fiber diet actually raises the age of puberty to a more appropriate age, one might wonder what effect it might have on social problems such as teenage pregnancy. But the bottom line is that diet is likely to be very important in breast cancer risk.

Protein and Protein Sources

Research has implicated animal proteins more than other sources of protein. One reason may be the tendency of chemicals such as DDT to concentrate in animal tissues. DDT is still commonly found in meats, years after it was banned. Is this a serious problem in terms of cancer risk?

"It's a very reasonable question," Alabaster said. "I don't think we have the evidence one way or another at the moment. But certainly if you're trying to minimize your risk, you're going to identify risk factors, some of which may be well-established, while others are theoretical. As Immanuel Kant said, 'It is often necessary to make a decision on the basis of knowledge sufficient for action but insufficient to satisfy the intellect.' I think we have to act on our best information. Put the question the other way around: If you know that animal food sources

"If you know that animal food sources contain a lot of these substances which you know are potentially harmful, it doesn't make a whole lot of sense to go on eating them."

Dr. Oliver Alabaster

contain a lot of these substances which you know are potentially harmful, it doesn't make a whole lot of sense to go on eating them."

Vitamins, Minerals, and Free Radicals

Micronutrients are parts of the diet that are required in only very small amounts: vitamins, minerals, and trace elements. They just might be the David that can slay the Goliath of cancer. To see how they work, we need to take a look at how cancer develops.

As a normal part of body chemistry, molecules called *free radicals* are produced, which can damage the DNA in our cells. Evidence suggests that this damage may lead to cancer. Compounds which block the effects of free radicals may help prevent cancer. "Free radicals are like a terrorist group that tours around creating havoc," Alabaster said. "They are highly unstable molecules. The hypothesis is that in their search for stability, they actually end up attacking cellular DNA. They may damage the DNA in such a way that the cell is transformed into a cancer cell."

Happily, there are foods which can neutralize the free radicals which have formed. These are called antioxidants. Beta-carotene, vitamins C and E, and the mineral selenium all have antioxidant properties. These compounds can neutralize free radicals and potentially limit the damage that contributes to cancer and possibly to aging and heart disease as well.

Beta-carotene occurs naturally in dark green, yellow, and orange vegetables. In the body, beta-carotene becomes vitamin A. Researchers at the National Cancer Institute are finding that beta-carotene and vitamin A help protect against cancer. For example, asbestos workers, particularly those who smoke, are at tremendous risk for lung cancer. But they are protected somewhat when their diet includes foods rich in beta-carotene.

"Up until now," says NCI's Peter Greenwald, "we really haven't been able to do anything for those people except to tell them not to smoke. We don't have a good means of early detection for lung cancer. So the study aims to see if we can prevent the onset of cancer." Studies of this type showed significant benefits from beta-carotene and vitamin A. "There are over twenty epidemiological studies," Greenwald said. "These studies show that populations having diets high in beta-carotene or vitamin A have lower cancer rates. I do want to emphasize that smokers still would be at a tremendously high risk of lung cancer, and they should stop smoking. They should not hold their breath in the hope that beta-carotene or vitamin A will prevent lung cancer, even if it somewhat lowers risk. People should not feel they're safe from cancer if they take a vitamin pill."

If your diet includes a generous amount of whole grain cereals or breads, a variety of dark green and yellow vegetables, beans, and fruits, you will be tapping the best sources of beta-carotene, vitamins C and E, and selenium. In addition, these foods contribute fiber, which is also very important.

In spite of our best efforts, free radicals will do some DNA damage. Fortunately, the body has another line of defense. It can actually repair damaged DNA. To do so, it needs folic acid, a B vitamin found in dark green leafy vegetables, fruits, wheat germ, dried peas and beans, and other foods. Human experiments have shown that folic acid helps repair chromosomal damage, as Alabaster relates. "Folic acid has been found in human experiments to protect cells against damage by powerful mutagens, such as caffeine. A mutagen like caffeine causes breaks at fragile sites in chromosomes. The fragile sites that are susceptible to mutagens are also the sites that have been found to be damaged in virtually all human solid tumors. If you take human volunteers and load them up with a high dose of folic acid and then give them the mutagen, you get no damage to the chromosomes. The implication of this work is that a diet rich in folic acid should optimize your DNA repair pathways, limiting the damage of carcinogens.

> *"Smokers should not hold their breath in the hope that beta-carotene or vitamin A will prevent lung cancer, even if it somewhat lowers risk. People should not feel they're safe from cancer if they take a vitamin pill."*
>
> **Dr. Peter Greenwald**

"So if you used antioxidants to inhibit free radical damage in the first place and folic acid to enhance repair in the second place,"Alabaster said, "you may end up with more stable cells."

There are other cancer-fighting micronutrients as well. Cruciferous vegetables, that is, broccoli, cauliflower, Brussels sprouts, and cabbage contain natural chemicals called *indoles* and *aromatic isothiocyanates*, which help prevent cancer. Garlic and onions contain large quantities of *quercetin*, a natural chemical which appears to have anti-cancer properties. In China, people who consume large quantities of garlic and onions (about three ounces a day) have less than half the risk of stomach cancer compared to those who consume only an ounce per day of these vegetables.

What are the best bets? Vegetables are essential. Dark green and yellow vegetables supply beta-carotene and vitamin C. The cruciferous vegetables contribute indoles and isothyocyanates. Whole grains in cereals and breads contribute vitamin E and selenium. And vegetables, fruits, grains, and beans supply fiber and are naturally low in fat.

A New Dietary Balance

"The fact that chemical pollution is responsible for a relatively small percentage of cancer cases and diet and

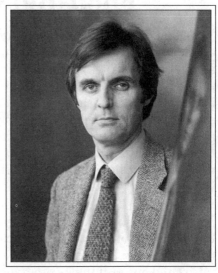

Dr. Oliver Alabaster

smoking are responsible for 70-80 percent suggests that the bulk of cancer can be modified by decisions we make ourselves," Alabaster said. "We don't have to wait for the federal government to do something. We can actually do something right now. The basic message that should be conveyed is that at least 70 percent of cancer is thought to be preventable based on what we now know. That is an astonishing figure which I would never have guessed at five years ago."

Chapter 4

Uninvited Guests: Food-Borne Illness

That "FLU" you had last winter may not have been the "flu" at all. It may have come from your supermarket's poultry department—one out of three chickens in the retail store carries live infectious salmonella bacteria. Or it might have come from a hamburger or a carton of eggs. Poultry, meat, and eggs at the supermarket have become "surprise packages," containing an unpredictable variety of contaminants: DDT and other pesticides, hormones, antibiotics, and live bacteria and other organisms that may cause millions of cases of "flu"-like illness every year in the U.S.

We like to think of our food products as coming to us in pristine packages produced under immaculate conditions, carefully monitored by trained government inspectors. Unfortunately, this is hardly the case. Take poultry, for example: modern farm operations raise chickens as if they were popcorn. A few thousand tiny chicks are put into a large steel building, and the doors are closed. Eight weeks later, thousands of big, round, fluffy, white birds are shoulder-to-shoulder, ready to be sold to slaughter. Unlike popcorn, however, they have been producing excrement continuously. In the cramped factory-farm design, there is nowhere they can go to get out of it.

As Assistant Secretary of Agriculture, Carol Tucker Foreman was responsible for the meat inspection system during the Carter Administration. She was gravely concerned that consumers were being routinely sold meat products that contained contaminants of all sorts and that the government had done little to stop it.

"Chickens are dirty animals," Foreman said. "Turkeys are dirty animals. When they are raised in close confinement, any filth that they pick up is going to be transferred from one bird to another. There are thousands of birds in a chicken house. You can imagine, they just live on a bed of feces. Their droppings are all over the place. They peck at their own droppings. They peck at each other. To the extent they fall down they get covered with feces."

One might hope that chicken houses would be cleaned occasionally, but the cramped conditions of the modern chicken operation are more like a factory than a farm. No one could possibly sweep around the birds during the growing season.

"'Would you stand on your left leg please?'" Forman laughed. "If you pass by a chicken house in the summertime, you feel fairly confident that they don't clean them out very often. They clean the floor at the end of the raising of each flock, if then."

Most operations, in fact, clean their buildings only about once a year, so for their whole lives the chickens are walking through their accumulating excrement.

"They're then brought to the slaughterhouse." Foreman said. "Chickens are hung upside down and slaughtered, and then their feathers are beaten and hosed off. The beating process that dislodges the feathers tends to beat into the skin of the chicken any feces or other dirt that they happen to have on them. So instead of getting it off, it's beaten in."

A former executive director of the Consumer Federation of America, Carol Tucker Foreman came from Arkansas with a good-natured directness and an uncompromising demand for safety. Her description of the disease-ridden meat industry is reminiscent of

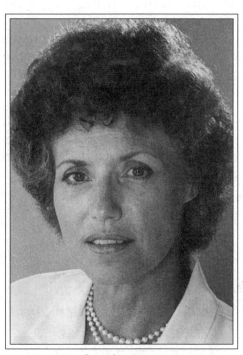

Carol Tucker Foreman

Upton Sinclair's classic condemnation of the Chicago slaughter-houses, *The Jungle*. Chickens not already covered with salmonella are likely to be contaminated as they go through the slaughterhouse.

"You have a production line that's run at a very rapid speed," Foreman said. "The chickens are eviscerated. If you've got real fancy equipment, you can run the line very, very fast and never puncture an intestine. But if your equipment is a little old or isn't adjusted just right, you'll puncture the intestines on large numbers of birds, and then the feces contaminate the birds.

"The last big place in the line where they get that contamination is when they put the poultry through a water bath. After all, it's a dead bird. It's a warm animal. In order to keep it from spoiling, you have to reduce its temperature very rapidly. They put it into a bath of very cold water. Any filth that's on the bird gets put into the bath water.

"Under the USDA rules, if there are feces on a bird, you can use all the meat if you wash the bird with chlorinated water. These days I would probably require both cutting [off the contaminated part] and washing because the salmonella level is too high. It's not enough to say that a particular process doesn't increase the contamination level. You ought to be looking for a process that decreases it.

"The Germans and the Common Market countries have now begun requiring a spin-drum process. American producers don't want to do that for a variety of reasons, not the least of which is that chickens are very absorbent animals. When you put them into the water bath to chill them they gain a little weight. Since chicken is sold by the pound, over a period of time it's a substantial financial difference to the company. The average broiler is about four pounds. If you can add a quarter of a pound or an eighth of a pound in water pickup, that's very important to the economics of the industry."

The water and juice in chicken packages has been called "fecal soup." It is often loaded with disease-causing salmonella and other bacteria. Why doesn't inspection pick up the bacterial contamination? Because salmonella bacteria are not visible to the naked eye.

> *"People have gone to the store and picked up packages of poultry and taken them off to a laboratory and checked them for salmonella contamination. The number of birds contaminated has been shown in several studies to be around a third."*
>
> **Carol Tucker Foreman**

"You can't see salmonella," Foreman said. "Inspection is done in a horse-and-buggy way. There are four billion chickens slaughtered each year, and each one of them is examined by a warm human being. They take a bird and they kind of feel a leg and a wing at the same time, and they look at the back, and they turn it and look at the front, and then they tilt it and look into the body cavity and feel the viscera. Inspectors look for obvious filth, for abscesses and tumors, and for broken bones, which I've never been sure is terribly important to consumers. They place a high premium on having a plant that's clean and a bird that looks good at the end of the line. Only one or two diseases that make chickens sick cause humans to be ill. But because poultry inspection was initially intended for the improvement of the animal stock, those were the things that inspectors concentrated on. You can't see salmonella. You can see things like feces that you assume are associated with it, but you can't see the salmonella. It may be much more extensive than any filth you can see.

As the chicken is packaged and sent to the supermarket, it carries the live salmonella along. Studies have looked at how often chicken is contaminated with salmonella. "The number of birds contaminated by salmonella has been shown in several studies to be around a third," Foreman said. "The people have gone to the store and picked up packages of poultry and taken them off to a laboratory and checked them for salmonella contamination. About a third."

> *"One of the big reasons that the incidence of salmonella poisoning in the United States is increasing these days is that we eat a lot more chicken than we used to."*
>
> **Carol Tucker Foreman**

Can the customer know that a certain brand of chicken is safe? Foreman remarked, "No, because if you went to the store and checked you would find salmonella contamination in any of the famous brands. Until we know more about preventing salmonella contamination and until the way USDA does inspection is changed, the public will have to be very, very careful about how they handle chicken.

"One of the big reasons that the incidence of salmonella poisoning in the United States is increasing these days is that we eat a lot more chicken than we used to," Foreman said. "We eat a lot of it in delicatessen settings. Making chicken salad in a mass operation is an invitation to salmonella. You put mayonnaise and chicken together with a little salmonella in it, and if the temperature gets a bit too high, you're going to have an enormous multiplication of the bacteria."

Salmonella illness often masquerades as the "flu," with vomiting, diarrhea, crampy abdominal pain and low-grade fever. It begins within 6 to 48 hours after ingestion of contaminated food. Usually, the illness passes within several days without treatment, but sometimes it persists and becomes very serious. It may spread through the blood to infect the bones, joints, lungs, liver, kidney, or the membranes that surround the heart and brain. And in thousands of cases each year, it is fatal.

"It is a significant problem," said Mitchell Cohen, M.D., of the Centers for Disease Control in Atlanta. The CDC is the focal point where information on contagious illnesses is gathered and from which investigations into outbreaks are directed. They have found that the reported cases of salmonella are only the tip of the iceberg.

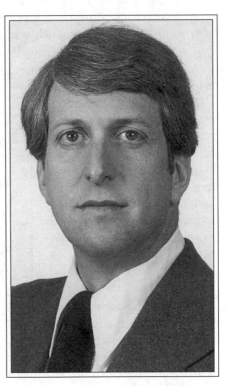

Dr. Mitchell Cohen

"It's been estimated that salmonellosis costs patients and producers over a billion dollars each year," Cohen said, "and that the reported cases only represent one-tenth to one-hundredth of the actual number of cases. There are probably between 400,000 and four million cases of salmonellosis a year in the United States."

Who should be concerned? The high fever, diarrhea, meningitis, infections of bones, joints, and the blood that can occur from salmonella illness are not treats for anyone. It can be quite serious, especially among the elderly. But there is another group at even more risk, the highest incidence being in three-month-old babies. All too often, diarrhea and fever in infants is caused by salmonella.

Of course, small babies do not eat chicken. How do they get salmonella? Raw meat can pass infectious bacteria onto any surface it touches. A mother may wipe up chicken juice from the counter top and later wipe off her baby's pacifier with the same sponge. The pacifier goes in the baby's mouth along with the infectious salmonella bacteria. Or simply touching raw chicken or other meat can pass bacteria which can survive on the hands for several hours. Salmonella can also infect an adult and then be passed to a child. "Cross-contamination is the most serious problem with salmonella," Foreman said. "If you open a package of chicken on the counter and pick the pieces out, there's always some water and meat juice in the bottom of the container. You cut the chicken up on a cutting board, a wooden cutting board for example, and then wipe the counter clean with a sponge and toss the sponge into the sink. Salmonella just love a sponge. And then they get passed on to the tabletop or to utensils or to anything else that you might use the sponge on. Or you may use that cutting board to cut up vegetables."

Cohen adds, "It's likely that the organisms are brought into the household, for example, through contaminated chicken, and are transferred to food preparation surfaces or utensils and eventually to the infant's formula. There also can be direct transmission to an infant from a person who has been infected. Salmonellosis in the very young or old can be a very serious illness."

> *"We have had outbreaks of salmonella related to almost every food of animal origin: poultry, beef, pork, eggs, milk, and milk products."*
>
> **Dr. Mitchell Cohen**

All this from bringing chicken into the household? Salmonella is not only found in chickens. Any animal product can be contaminated, as Dr. Cohen points out. "We have had outbreaks of salmonella related to almost every food of animal origin: poultry, beef, pork, eggs, milk, and milk products."

Salmonella can even get inside an egg. Again, the problem is the intensely crowded conditions of the modern factory-farm, where chickens literally live in each others feces. In the 1960s, egg products used in baking frequently caused outbreaks of disease. It also became clear that salmonella on the surface of an egg could get inside if the shell were cracked. But there have been increasing reports of intact grade A eggs harboring live salmonella, causing thousands of cases of illness. The bacteria pass into the eggs while still inside the chicken, and evidently can also pass through the shell from external contamination.

"People have to appreciate that there are certain high-risk food items," Cohen said. "Foods of animal origin are likely to be contaminated with salmonella."

All animal products are potential sources of salmonella. Steps that can help prevent salmonella infection are detailed at the end of this chapter.

The Antibiotic Connection

Cattle, chickens, and other animals often carry salmonella and other bacteria in their intestinal tracts. Farmers now routinely aggravate this problem by feeding low doses of antibiotics to their animals. The farmer is not using the antibiotics to kill off invading bacteria. The doses farmers use are *subtherapeutic*, that is, insufficient to counter infections. The antibiotics are used to make the animals grow faster, increasing the farmer's profit margin. For reasons no one fully understands, antibiotics promote the growth of the animals. In the process, they foster the growth of bacteria that can resist antibiotics. New strains of bacteria develop in these animals, strains that are very hard to control. When they infect animals or people, our usual antibiotics may be entirely ineffective.

> *"A quarter or more of salmonella are now resistant to commonly used antibiotics."*
>
> **Dr. Mitchell Cohen**

Antibiotics in livestock feeds have given bacteria the upper hand in human illness. If antibiotic-resistant salmonella are eaten in food, they can remain dormant in the intestinal tract, held in check by the normal intestinal bacteria. But if antibiotics are then used for some other condition, they will kill off the normal gut bacteria that had held the salmonella in check. The salmonella can resist the antibiotics, and then overgrow and cause a very serious illness.

"A quarter or more of salmonella are now resistant to commonly used antibiotics," Cohen said. "In a recent report, a person died because she was treated with what was thought to be the drug of choice. The organism was subsequently found to be resistant to that antibiotic."

Because the indiscriminate use of antibiotics promotes the growth of resistant bacteria, doctors now avoid using antibiotics unless clearly necessary. But antibiotics are a routine ingredient in animal agriculture.

"If you go to your pediatrician or your internist with a little sore throat," Foreman said, "they don't give you penicillin until they're sure it's a bacterial and not a viral infection. They don't want to overuse penicillin. And yet two-thirds or three-quarters of all of the penicillin and tetracycline manufactured in this country go for subtherapeutic use in animal production. As a matter of course, poultry, cattle, and hogs in this country are raised on feed that is medicated. American Cyanamid doesn't make its profits selling antibiotics for human beings; they make it selling antibiotics for animals."

In 1977, the Food and Drug Administration proposed eliminating the subtherapeutic use of penicillin and tetracycline in animal feed. But just as the sympathies for farmers have led Congress to subsidize tobacco crops and dairy products, Congress also has not allowed restrictions on antibiotics used to promote animal growth.

E. coli

In January, 1993, food poisoning reached a new and grotesque level. That was the beginning of the Jack-in-the-Box disaster. A new bacterium, called E. coli 0157:H7, had caused its first disease outbreak 11 years earlier, soon followed by several others. E. coli is found in cow feces. During slaughter and processing, it contaminates meat and is undetected by government meat inspectors, who check only the appearance of meat and do not routinely use bacterial tests. On January 10, 1993, a two-year-old-boy in Tacoma, Washington, ate a cheeseburger at a Jack-in-the-Box restaurant. The next day he developed fever and vomiting. On January 13, he was hospitalized. Nine days later, he was dead.

The Jack-in-the-Box restaurant chain in several western states sold ground beef that looked and tasted normal, but made 600 children and adults seriously ill. Hospitalization was necessary for 144 of them. Three children and one adult died.

The U.S. Department of Agriculture rushed in. Secretary Mike Espy and others held hearings, promising aggressive new programs. But it soon became clear the Department of Agriculture's main interest was not in cleaning up meat products, but rather in cleaning up the image of American agriculture, while brushing aside consumer worries. A year later, virtually nothing had been done to correct the problem. And on January 8, 1994, a thirteen-year-old boy in Aberdeen, Washington, had a burger at a fast food restaurant. Fifteen days later he was dead. His parents thought the E. coli problem must have been solved, because the government had seemingly given it so much attention. But they learned a bitter lesson. The government is doing virtually nothing to stop it Federal officials estimate there may be as many as 20,000 cases of E. coli infection every year.

E. coli 0517:H7 infections come mainly from beef and raw milk, and from water contaminated by animal wastes. Like salmonella, it is easily transmitted by kitchen surfaces and utensils, and by person-to-person contact. Illness is caused, not by the bacterium itself, but by a toxin it produces. Symptoms range from mild diarrhea to severe cramps with bloody diarrhea. Some cases progress to the hemolytic uremic syndrome (HUS) in which the bacterial toxin destroys blood cells and platelets, and damages the kidneys and other organs. About five to ten percent of those with HUS die. Current antibiotics and antimotility drugs are useless against E. coli 0157:H7 and may even worsen the disease.

A Department of Agriculture survey tested beef carcasses between October, 1992, and November, 1993. Disease-causing bacteria, including clostridia, campylobacter, staphylococci, listeria, salmonella, and, yes, E. coli 0157:H7, were found on 15 percent of them.[1] There is no reason to expect this problem to get better any time soon, and it is yet another reason to steer clear of animal products.

DDT and Other Three-Letter Words

All sorts of chemicals find their way into foods. Our inspectors do not have ways of checking for them all. But even for those that can be detected, however, the foods are rarely removed from the market. The monitoring process does not generally report on samples until after the remaining foods have been sold and consumed. "You may find out two weeks later that it was just laden with DDT," Foreman said. "By that time the meat's been eaten."

DDT is not used in this country any more. It was banned in 1972, although sporadic use of the chemical continued in the next few years. But DDT remains in the environment. Since its widespread use as a sprayed pesticide, it circulates widely in the atmosphere. As it settles on the soil it becomes part of plants and, particularly, of animals who concentrate the chemical in their fatty tissues. Is DDT still found in meat?

"Sure," Foreman said. "It's one of the residues that they find most frequently. DDT is ubiquitous. Once it's in the atmosphere, it stays there for a very long time. If there's ground that's contaminated with DDT, the corn grown or stored near that ground comes out contaminated with DDT and the animals may be contaminated with it."

In addition, chemicals banned for use in this country can, in some cases, continue to be manufactured for export. Agricultural products which are then imported into the U.S. may carry these chemicals back into our food supply.

PCBs

Polychlorinated biphenyls (PCBs) were manufactured for use in electrical transformers and other commercial applications. From this humble beginning, PCBs have achieved notoriety as some of the most poisonous chemicals ever produced.

PCBs cause cancer. Acute exposure can cause liver damage and a variety of other symptoms. PCBs are easily passed from a nursing mother to her breast-fed infant.

Although manufacture of the chemicals was banned in 1979, getting rid of them continues to be a major problem. PCBs have often been found in fish, as a result of leakage or intentional dumping of PCBs into waterways. A 1987 study, conducted by Laval University in Quebec, showed that Eskimo women have PCB concentrations in their breast milk that are more than double the tolerance levels set by the Canadian government. These concentrations are sufficient to cause serious illnesses in their nursing infants. The cause is the fish-based Eskimo diet. PCBs can spread many, many miles from the dumping site. Researchers at Wayne State University in Detroit found that women eating Lake Michigan fish only two or three times per month gave birth to children who were sluggish, had smaller head circumferences and lower birth weights compared to the children of mothers who ate less (or no) fish. "I would advise women of child-bearing age not to eat fatty fish like salmon and lake trout at all," said Joseph L. Jacobsen, one of the Wayne State researchers. The problem was PCBs passed from the fish to the women who ate them. PCBs can remain in the body for prolonged periods of time, a stock-pile of toxins waiting to damage a developing baby. Birds, such as ducks and geese, that feed on these fish may also be highly contaminated. In addition, PCB contamination of animal feeds has spread the chemical to meats and eggs.

Chemicals on Fruits and Vegetables

Unlike the chemical contaminants in meats or milk which are permeated throughout the product, the chemicals on produce are usually on the surface. Peeling fruits and vegetables is often helpful. All produce should be washed. A dilute soap solution and plenty of water will help remove some chemical residues. Waxes cannot be washed off, and waxed produce should be peeled.

When buying produce, ask for organically grown produce. Most health food stores carry a good selection. Avoid non-domestic produce, since it may have been treated with chemicals now banned in the U.S. Of course, some people grow vegetables of their own.

Thanks, But No Thanks

As problematic as chemical residues on produce may be, chemicals in meats are even more difficult to deal with. These chemicals cannot be washed or peeled from meats as they sometimes can from produce.

Meats must be regarded as carrying live infectious bacteria, parasites, and chemical residues. Although both Foreman and Cohen believe that correct handling and cooking can minimize the chances that bacteria or parasites will survive in the kitchen, bringing these products into the home always poses a risk of contamination.

The surest way to avoid chemical contamination is to decline the dubious honor of being at the top of the food chain. If plants contain a low-level of chemical contamination, animals who eat them will concentrate these chemicals. If these animals are, in turn, eaten by others (or by humans), a progressive increase in the level of contamination occurs. By choosing plant foods, we find less contamination.

At the very top of the food chain is the human infant. The breast-fed infant is the target, not only of the contamination ingested by his or her mother, but of her tendency to further concentrate chemicals in her fatty tissues, such as breast tissue. According to a study at Colorado State University, published in the *New England Journal of Medicine*, vegetarian mothers have far lower levels of chemical contaminants in their breast milk than non-vegetarians.[2] The more our diet relies on foods from plants, rather than from animals, the less contamination we will encounter. The more we know about the foods we eat, the better able we will be to protect ourselves.

Chapter 5

Other Common Health Problems

Are varicose veins, appendicitis, or gallstones related to what we eat? Believe it or not, the answer is yes. Surprising links are being found between dietary factors and many common health problems. Constipation, hemorrhoids, hiatus hernia, diabetes, osteoporosis, kidney disease, and even impotence are among the other common problems related to foods. In this chapter, we will take a brief look at these connections. The story begins, not in the United States, but in Africa.

Denis Burkitt and Fiber

For 20 years, Denis Burkitt, M.D., practiced surgery in Africa. An adventurous and widely traveled man, Burkitt achieved fame in medicine for identifying and curing a form of childhood cancer now known as Burkitt's lymphoma, the first human cancer shown to be caused by a virus (see Chapter 3).

On the heels of this important work, Burkitt began to notice that many common Western diseases were conspicuous by their absence in Africa. For example, while there might be two cases of appendicitis a day in the major hospitals of Western countries, Burkitt found only about two cases *per year* among Africans. Many other illnesses were also extraordinarily rare wherever modern food preparation methods had not been put to use.

"I was doing ward rounds in English hospitals and American hospitals," Burkitt said, "and it struck me that all the beds were full of patients suffering from diseases I didn't see in Africa: coronary heart disease, the commonest cause of death; gallstones, the commonest abdominal operation; appendicitis, the commonest abdominal emergency; varicose veins and hemorrhoids, the commonest venous disorders; colorectal cancer, the second commonest cancer death; diverticular disease, one of the commonest disorders of the gut; hiatus hernia, one of the commonest disorders of the stomach. It seems as if we have in front of us the mass of disease, which has to be preventable. I said to myself, if it really is possible to prevent our common diseases, why are we spending our time treating them?"

He took an interest in the hypothesis of a retired naval physician named Captain Cleave that many diseases common to Western countries were the result of overly refined foods, especially sugar and white flour. While Cleave had only found a piece of the puzzle, it was enough to get Burkitt going.

Burkitt came to find that refined sugar was by no means the whole explanation. A critical factor is fiber. In the modern refining methods used for grains, the fiber—the portion of vegetable foods that resists digestion—is discarded. In the process, the fiber content of the diet drops dramatically. At the same time, vegetables, beans, and fruits have become second-class foods, while meat and dairy products have become a larger and larger part of our routine. As the high-fat, low-fiber diet takes hold around the world, Africa, India, and Asian countries that have never known Western diseases see an increasing occurrence of epidemics of diabetes, obesity, appendicitis, colon cancer, and heart disease following successively like a funeral procession.

Burkitt was not the first person to be interested in fiber. Hippocrates used whole grains as medical treatments. The Kellogg brothers in America had been proponents of the health benefits of cereal grains.

"And there was an interesting chap in the 1920s called Arbuthnot Lane," Burkitt said. "He was a surgeon. And he got the concept that most ills were due to stagnation of the fecal content in the colon. So being a surgeon, he thought the best thing to do was to cut out the colon. He thought it would be a good thing if all children had their colons cut out early in life, and then they would be exempt from all sorts of problems! He cut out the colon for all kinds of conditions. And then he suddenly came to the conclusion that it was much easier to give bran than to cut out the colon, and it had the same effect. So he gave up cutting out the colon and gave people bran instead."

As cultures undergo a Westernization of diet—for example, Japanese or Africans coming to America, or Asians adopting a Western diet within their own countries—diseases emerge in a certain order. Some are seen very soon; others only after many years. Interestingly, these diseases appear in the changing population in about the same order as they develop in individuals. For example, obesity becomes evident well before heart attacks.

"Diabetes is unknown in undomesticated animals," Burkitt said. "It's the commonest endocrine disease in Western man, and it's one of the first diseases that comes in after a change in life-style.

Obesity comes in early. Appendicitis not quite so early, probably a decade or two later. But we've never seen gallstones or coronary heart disease emerge until about thirty years after diabetes becomes common. You never find coronary heart disease in a culture without diabetes.

> *"Diabetes is the commonest endocrine disease in Western man, and it's one of the first diseases that comes in after a change in lifestyle."*
>
> **Denis Burkitt**

"After the second World War, the government helped to feed the Pima Indians of Arizona," Burkitt said. "They suddenly plunged into popcorn, french fries, and hamburgers. They have the highest rate of gallstones in the world now and the second highest rate of diabetes, after the people on the island of Nauru who suddenly became millionaires overnight and changed their whole life-style." The traditional diet of the these Indians—desert legumes, with occasional cacti, fish, and seeds—has been shown to be superior from a health perspective than the foods the government has unloaded on them.[1] Meanwhile, in parts of rural Africa where a Westernized diet has not yet taken hold, these chronic diseases are still rare. Childhood illnesses, particularly infections, do occur, but the Western diet-related diseases are very uncommon. As a result, many adult Africans live to a ripe old age.

"In a total community survey in South Africa, when they took blacks and whites relative to their numbers in the community, it was amazing—they found sixteen times as many centenarians amongst the blacks as amongst the whites. Lots of people think you don't get old blacks. There are lots of old blacks. Those who are 45 or 50 have a statistically better chance of getting to eighty than white people have. They're not going to die of coronary heart disease or lung cancer or bowel cancer or these things."

So while an American is more likely to survive infancy, he or she is far more likely to be killed by the diseases of mid-life. And the reason is diet. "All of these diseases really are manifestations of maladaptation to a new environment," Burkitt said. "Western man has made more change in his diet over the last six or eight generations—150 to 200 years—than man has made throughout the whole of his sojourn on earth. We have suddenly plunged into an environment to which we are not adapted. Our bodies are the same as Stone Age bodies genetically, anatomically, physiologically, and everything else. But what we put into them is quite different. We are putting supermarket food into Stone Age bodies. In lectures I often use a picture of a Stone Age man with a club over his shoulder pushing a trolley into a supermarket. We're not adapted. It's no good saying let's wait until we adapt because that might take another ten thousand years. The only thing we can do is to go back a bit."

> *"Western man has made more change in his diet over the last six or eight generations-150 to 200 years-than man has made throughout the whole of his sojourn on earth."*
>
> **Dr. Denis Burkitt**

We need to bring back the fiber—that is, unrefined plant foods, particularly grains and legumes. We also need to cut back on the meats, dairy products, and fried foods—the high-fat fare, devoid of fiber and carbohydrate, that has insinuated its way into our diet.

"I first thought fiber was almost the whole thing," Burkitt said. "Now I recognize it's a question of fiber, starch, fat, salt, and sugar. They all play a role. Cleave would never accept that fat played a role, and he died of atherosclerosis himself a few years ago."

Constipation

The refining of grains has led, over the last two centuries, to the gradual disappearance of fiber from the diet. Whole wheat bread has been replaced by soft white bread. Other whole grains find no place in the diet of modern Western countries. In the digestive tract, fiber holds water, which keeps the intestinal contents soft. Without fiber to hold water, digestion compacts the intestinal contents, which then move only very slowly. As a result, constipation has become almost a routine in the modern world.

"It has been said very authoritatively that if we got the fiber back in our diet, the whole of the laxative industry would be in liquidation within six months," Burkitt said. "Because fiber holds water. The only reason you have a laxative industry is because you've taken fiber out of your diet. And I mean cereal fiber. Never kid yourself that you're getting much fiber by eating salad. Americans eat more salad than any nation on Earth, and they're the most constipated nation on the globe. So it doesn't help them at all. It's got to be cereal fiber. Beans are also good. Cabbage might help you a little bit, but fruit and green vegetables by and large are not much help from the point of view of constipation.

"The only reason you have a laxative industry is because you've taken fiber out of your diet."

Dr. Denis Burkitt

"Until a hundred years ago there was no cold storage and no canning. There was no way of storing food. The human race was adapted to live on what you could store on the floor of the barn. Those were cereals, whether it be wheat, rye, or others; legumes: peas and beans; millets and tubers: potatoes, carrots, turnips, and so on. Those are the things which we are no longer eating. We've thrown out our potatoes, and we've thrown out our bread."

The cure for constipation? Whole grains, such as wheat, oatmeal, and brown rice, and beans and other legumes in generous portions. When these are part of the daily diet, regularity follows.

Varicose Veins, Hemorrhoids, and Hiatus Hernia

As a result of the constipation that occurs on a fiber-depleted diet, straining to pass stools is a daily occurrence. Over the long run, this daily battle with constipation leads to other problems. The increase in pressure in the abdomen caused by straining is implicated as a cause of varicose veins, hemorrhoids, and hiatal hernia, as Burkitt explains:

"When you strain at stool, you put very high pressures in your abdominal cavity," Burkitt said. "These pressures are immediately transmitted to the veins draining the lower limbs. The pressures are held back at the first set of valves in the leg veins. Now it has been shown that the valves in the leg give way sequentially one after the other from above down. When all the valves are incompetent, gravity plus straining can make pressures in the veins of the lower part of the leg nearly as high as the blood pressures in arteries."

Under these pressures, veins are damaged. Varicose veins can result. Other evidence also indicates that abdominal straining can cause varicose veins. "People in Southeast Asia who ride tri-shaws struggle along with a couple of people sitting in front. They have far more varicose veins than people who stand all day cutting hair. People who climb the Himalayas carrying heavy loads tend to get varicose veins. Now these are consistent with straining as one cause." They are straining the abdomen and pushing blood down into the veins of the leg. Straining to pass stools does precisely the same thing.

Burkitt hypothesizes that hemorrhoids are caused by the same mechanism. Hemorrhoids are engorgements of normal blood vessels. Just as the veins of the legs distend under pressure, the hemorrhoidal vessels do the same thing. Repeated straining of the abdomen to pass stools forces blood to engorge the hemorrhoidal vessels. The solution is to make stools easier to pass. This is where fiber works: It retains water so that stools pass easily. Constipation is prevented and straining is unnecessary.

Increased pressures in the abdomen may also contribute to hiatus (or hiatal) hernia. Hiatus hernia is a condition in which part of the stomach is pushed upward through the diaphragm into the chest cavity. It typically causes no symptoms, but may contribute to heartburn for some patients.

"My hypothesis for hiatus hernia is beginning to be accepted by gastroenterologists," Burkitt said. "If you take a tennis ball and cut a hole in it and fill it with water and squeeze the tennis ball, the water goes out through the hole. Now, your abdominal cavity is the tennis ball. And every time you squeeze your tennis ball to void constipated stools you force the stomach out through the hole in the diaphragm which transmits the esophagus. Now, we have never found any community in the world which passes large soft stools and gets hiatus hernia."

> *"Never kid yourself that you're getting much fiber by eating salad. Americans eat more salad than any nation on Earth, and they're the most constipated nation on the globe."*
>
> **Dr. Denis Burkitt**

For these conditions, medical teaching has often ignored the causative role of dietary factors. "If you look in a textbook it will say that varicose veins are due to pregnancies or large abdominal tumors or standing. That's rubbish. It's just totally denied by the evidence," Burkitt said. "Total community surveys in North America have shown 50 percent of women over the age of 40 to have varicose veins. A recent study in New Guinea found only one varicose vein amongst 800 adult women. So how can you say that varicose veins are due to man not being adapted to the upright posture? We've had many surveys done in Africa and India. Most of them were under five percent.

"If you looked up the cause of hiatus hernia in our most popular surgical textbooks, it is said to be due to the lack of tone in the diaphragm with advancing age. But why is it that the diaphragm never lacks tone in Africa or India or the Middle East or Japan and only does in North America and Western Europe? This doesn't tell you anything, does it? Then it tells you it's due to large abdominal tumors, but a country with large abdominal tumors gets no hiatus hernia. Thirdly, it suggests it's due to pregnancy, when the countries with the most pregnancies have the least hiatus hernia. Fourthly, in an edition in the mid-1970s, it said 'women wearing corsets.' Well, how many women wear corsets?

"Again, if you have hypotheses which are totally at variance with evidence, you've got to scrap them, haven't you?"

Appendicitis

Appendicitis is rare in countries that have a high-fiber diet, according to numerous epidemiologic studies. In Uganda, Burkitt noticed that the only Africans who tended to develop appendicitis were those who had adopted Western dietary habits. He became wary about diagnosing appendicitis in Africans unless they could speak English, indicating their degree of contact with Western culture.

The appendix is a small, finger-like tube attached to the large intestine. It can become blocked by a small, compacted lump of stool. This blockage can lead to inflammation and infection, and characteristic abdominal pain. Removal of the appendix is then usually necessary.

Burkitt hypothesizes that the reason appendicitis is rare in countries maintaining traditional diets is that the fiber in their diet keeps stools soft, and so the appendix does not become blocked. If Westerners were to return the fiber to their diets, this common surgical emergency might become a medical rarity.

Fiber, Cholesterol, and Gallstones

Fiber helps lower cholesterol. Evidence shows that this is especially true of soluble fiber, such as oat bran. While this effect is partly due to the fact that high-fiber foods tend to displace high-fat foods from the menu, there may be other mechanisms involved. In the liver, cholesterol is turned into bile acids which are sent into the intestinal tract where they help in digestion. These bile acids can be reabsorbed and returned to the body's cholesterol pool. But fiber can trap bile acids in the intestinal tract and allow them to be excreted. This helps lower the cholesterol level in the blood.

This is obviously important in the prevention of heart disease. But there is another important benefit too: preventing gallstones. Cholesterol can form stones in the gallbladder. These stones can be the cause of persistent abdominal pain, and often lead to surgery. Removal of the gallbladder has become one of the commonest abdominal operations.

"There's a lot of evidence coming out now that fiber is protective against gallstones," Burkitt said. "If you feed volunteers high-fiber diets, you lower their cholesterol, and the bile has less of a tendency to form stones."

In addition, a high-fiber diet appears to increase the formation of a particular bile acid, called *chenodeoxycholate*, which has gallstone-dissolving properties. In combination with fiber's cholesterol-lowering effect, gallstones are much less likely to form.

"The great thing is we don't need to know these mechanisms in order to take action," Burkitt said. "It doesn't really matter what the mechanism is as long as you can demonstrate that a certain thing gives you the right results."

In America, gallbladder operations are an everyday event. In countries with a low-fat, high-fiber diet, they are rarely necessary. It is only those who adopt the diet of affluent countries who are at significant risk for the disease. "I only removed two gallbladders from Africans in my twenty years in Africa," Burkitt said. "One was a queen, one of the only two queens I ever operated on. So fifty percent of my gallstones were taken out of queens."

How much fiber should we actually be getting in our diet? "At the moment we are getting about twenty grams a day, in some parts of England only ten and some parts of America only ten. We ought to have a minimum of thirty grams, preferably forty, and it ought to be cereal fiber in particular. If we did only one thing in this country, if we multiplied our bread intake by two or three and never had it made from white flour, that would revolutionize the health of America."

The key factor, of course, is not to count the number of grams of fiber consumed each day, but rather to shift the diet so that healthy amounts of fiber, fat, and protein naturally fall into place.

This means a new emphasis on grains, legumes, vegetables, and fruits. As we do this, we will look better, feel better, and live free of many of the common problems that could otherwise take away the enjoyment of life.

Diabetes

In diabetes, the cells of the body cannot get the sugar they need. Glucose, a simple sugar, is the body's main fuel. It is present in the blood, but in diabetics it cannot get into the cells where it is needed. When diabetes starts in childhood, it is due to an inadequate supply of insulin, the hormone which ushers sugar into the cells of the body. Without insulin, the cell membranes keep sugar out. When diabetes begins in adulthood, it is not due to an inadequate supply of insulin. There is plenty of insulin in the blood stream, but the cells do not respond readily to it. Sugar cannot get into the cells, and it backs up in the blood stream. In the short run, diabetics may experience episodes of labored breathing, vomiting, and dehydration. In the long run, diabetics are at risk for heart disease, kidney problems, disorders of vision, and other difficulties.

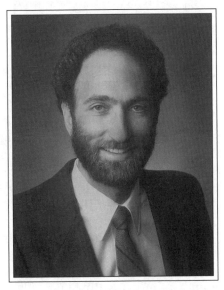

Dr. Monroe Rosenthal

The dietary approach to diabetes is illustrated by a treatment program that has been very helpful for people with the disease, called the Pritikin Program. The foundation of the program is not the ever-increasing regimen of medicines that has been the mainstay against diabetes over the last several decades, but, rather, replacing medicines as much as possible with low-fat foods and exercise.

Monroe Rosenthal, M.D., is the Medical Director of the Pritikin Program. Rosenthal is lean and athletic. When he is not working with patients to reverse the damage of years of bad diet at the Pritikin Center on the ocean front in Santa Monica, California, he can be found running marathons. He explains his approach to diabetes, "In the mid to late seventies, a popular belief was that since sugar is found in the urine of diabetics, that by not eating sugar or substances that are turned into sugar, such as starches, breads, fruit, and so forth, they would improve. This was really a misconception. When you take away the complex carbohydrates and refined sugars from the diet you're left with fat and protein."

Fat, in particular, is a problem for diabetics. The more fat there is in the diet, the harder time insulin has in getting sugar into the cell. Exactly how fat disables insulin's action is not clear. But what is clear is that minimizing fat helps insulin do its job much better. "By switching to a lower-fat diet," Rosenthal said, "whatever insulin is available seems to work more ef-fectively at incorporating sugar into the cells."

To reduce fat in the diet, the program drastically reduces meats, high-fat dairy products, and oils. At the same time, it increases grains, legumes, and vegetables. One study found that 21 of 23 patients on oral medications and 13 of 17 patients on insulin were able to get off their medication after 26 days on the program.[2] At two- and three-year follow-ups, most diabetics treated with this regimen have retained their gains.[3] The dietary changes are simple, but profound, and they work.

But there is a second essential component to managing diabe-tes. Through regular exercise, the need for insulin injections can often be reduced, and oral medications often become unnecessary. "An aerobic exercise program will allow sugar to enter the cells without the use of insulin," Rosenthal said. "This holds true not only for the adult patients but also to some extent for insulin-dependent juvenile diabetics. Exercising muscles have a voracious appetite for fuel. When an individual is engaged in regular aerobic exercise, the sugar is able to enter the cells without the need for as much, or any, insulin. The cells just sort of suck up the circulating sugar.

"We see many individuals who are on insulin because they're overweight, not exercising, and eating a lot of refined sugar and fat. Through diet and regular aerobic exercise, we can essentially get them off insulin and off oral agents, and get them to normal blood sugar values."

While people with adult-onset diabetes can often eliminate medications when their weight is reduced and foods and exercise are better controlled, those with childhood-onset diabetes will always need a source of insulin. The causes of insulin-dependent (childhood-onset) diabetes remain elusive. Although genetic fac-tors may be responsible for a predisposition to diabetes, it may be that other factors, such as nutrition, determine whether diabetes actually develops. Recent studies have implicated milk consumption as a contributor.[4] When milk consumption patterns were examined across various countries, there was a very strong correlation with the incidence of insulin-dependent diabetes. Studies of diabetic patients suggest that milk proteins cause an autoimmune reaction in which the body mistakenly attacks its own insulin-producing cells.[5] Even so, a good diet and regular exercise can minimize the amount of insulin these diabetics require. This is especially important given their tendency toward complications. Heart disease and other blood vessel problems are much more common in diabetics. So it is doubly important to keep fit and to keep fats in the diet to a minimum.

Rosenthal feels that diabetics are short-changed by the diets most doctors give them. "The typical American Diabetes Association diet is a diet high in fat. They limit the amount of butter, they cut down on eggs and so forth, but it still contains about 300 milligrams of cholesterol per day and around 30 per-cent fat. It's approaching our diet at a very tediously slow pace."

Problems with Protein:
Osteoporosis & Kidney Damage

Osteoporosis—the loss of bone tissue—is common in Western countries, particularly in women after menopause. Changes in diet and life-style may help prevent it. The key is not in milk or massive calcium supplements. Advertisements by the dairy industry notwithstanding, evidence shows that, beyond a certain minimum, eating calcium does little to help the body build bones.

> *"We have no evidence that osteoporosis has anything to do with calcuim intake, and there is very great doubt as to whether giving calcium has any effect on osteoporosis."*
>
> **Dr. Denis Burkitt**

"We have no evidence that osteoporosis has anything to do with calcium intake," Burkitt said, "and there is very great doubt as to whether giving calcium has any effect on osteoporosis."

Science magazine[6] on August 1, 1986, noted "the large body of evidence indicating no relationship between calcium intake and bone density." Dr. B. Lawrence Riggs of the Mayo Clinic measured bone densities and calcium intake in women for several years. He reported, "We found no correlation at all between calcium intake and bone loss, not even a trend." Some studies have found an effect of calcium intake on the density of the wrist bones, but little or no effect where it counts—the spine and hip.

What causes osteoporosis? First of all, hormones play a major role. After menopause, hormonal changes foster the loss of bone. Doctors often prescribe hormone supplements to women for precisely this reason. Such treatments are helpful in delaying osteoporosis, although their overall health risk remains controversial. But this is only part of the story. Another major factor appears to be the damaging effect of a high-protein diet.[7-9]

> *"We have a population that eats a high-protein diet, they don't exercise much, they smoke. Those are really the main reasons for the epidemic of osteoporosis."*
>
> **Dr. Monroe Rosenthal**

"The literature indicates that a high-protein diet, which the American diet certainly is, contributes to the epidemic of osteoporosis," Rosenthal said. "We have a population that eats a high-protein diet, they don't exercise much, they smoke. Those are really the main reasons for the epidemic of osteoporosis."

An overly generous amount of protein in the diet depletes the body's calcium. When protein is taken in, some is used for the body's various needs. Some of the excess is changed to urea in the liver. Urea is a powerful diuretic. When urea and the amino acids, which are the building blocks of proteins, enter the kidneys, they cause the loss of water and the loss of important minerals as well. Calcium is one of the minerals that is washed away in this process. In addition, as proteins break down to amino acids which are absorbed into the blood stream, the blood becomes slightly more acidic. To neutralize this acidic effect, calcium is pulled from bone material. This ultimately leads to an increase in calcium excretion in the urine. So the more protein we take in beyond the amount we need, the more calcium we lose.

"Researchers have estimated that doubling the protein in the diet leads to a 50 percent increase in calcium loss in the urine," says physician and nutrition author John A. McDougall, M.D. Like the Pritikin Center, McDougall has found that dietary changes can be phenomenally success-ful in treating a variety of illnesses. He sees patients at the St. Helena Hospital in Deer Park, California, and appears frequently on radio and television programs. He is concerned about osteoporosis and the failure of most doctors to address its causes. Calcium supplements simply do not eliminate the loss of calcium caused by a high-protein diet.

> *"Reserachers have estimated that doubling the protein in the diet leads to a 50 percent increase in clacium loss in the urine."*
>
> **Dr. John McDougall**

"Calcium supplements are usually ineffective in compensating for this loss," McDougall said. "Studies of Eskimo populations have shown that their tremendous intake of fish protein is accompanied by significant osteoporosis. Eskimos over the age of 40 have an average of 10 to 15 percent less bone tissue than do comparable Caucasians in the U.S. The Eskimo diet includes a large quantity of fish bones, so they have a very high calcium intake, as high as 2500 milligrams a day. The damage done by their high-protein diet is not compensated for by all the calcium they consume."

Americans get into trouble not only with the amount of protein they eat but with the *type* of protein as well. "There are about 20 common amino acids that make up the different proteins," McDougall said. "Three of these contain the element sulfur in their chemical structure. These sulfur-containing amino acids have a strong calcium-depleting effect on the kidneys. Animal proteins have a higher content of these sulfur-containing amino acids than do vegetable proteins."

Meats, including poultry and fish, contain too much protein and too high a concentration of the sulfur-containing amino acids.

To prevent osteoporosis, we must also *use* our bones. Weight-bearing exercise helps build strong bones. In addition, we need to be aware that alcohol and tobacco aggravate bone loss. And keeping our protein intake to more modest levels is important.

The dairy industry, of course, is using osteoporosis as a marketing tool. They would like us to believe that the body's careful regulation of calcium absorption and bone structure can be tricked by simply ingesting a large amount of milk. "But it's not valid," Burkitt said. "People with quite low calcium intake get infinitely less osteoporosis."

McDougall adds another reason to avoid dairy products: the milk proteins often elicit allergic responses. "Dairy products are the most common cause of food allergies," McDougall said. "Look at all the allergic reactions to dairy products that have been noted in the scientific literature: canker sores, digestive problems, skin conditions, respiratory reactions, and so on." This is a separate problem from lactose intolerance, the inability to digest the milk

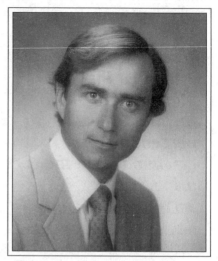

Dr. John McDougall

sugar, which causes indigestion in many Africans and Asians. Dairy allergy is a sensitivity to the milk proteins, and is often manifested in subtle ways, as McDougall points out, "People don't know until they get away from them for a while, and then try them again. And they say, 'Oh, that's why I had a stuffy nose all the time,' or 'That's why I have post-nasal drip.' That's why I try to get my patients to change completely. When people avoid dairy products completely, they often find improvement in symptoms which they did not realize were caused by milk proteins."

Milk consumption is also implicated as a contributor to cataracts. Although there are other factors, such as excessive exposure to sunlight, which contribute to opacities of the lens, it has been suggested that *galactose*, a breakdown product of the milk sugar *lactose*, may gradually damage the lens. Indeed, a detailed review of the subject published in 1982 showed that populations which consume large amounts of dairy products tend to have a much higher incidence of cataracts than populations which avoid dairy products.[10] Nursing children are better able to break down both lactose and galactose. But as children grow older, the capacity to metabolize these compounds diminishes. Many Caucasian adults can break down lactose well, but do not rapidly metabolize the galactose which comes from it. As a result, they are at risk for the problems which may be caused by high levels of galactose. The correlation between the use of dairy products and cataracts is real, but the cause-and-effect relationship is only theoretical, awaiting more observation.

> *"Dairy products are the most common cause of food allergies. When people avoid dairy products completely, they often find improvement in symptoms which they did not realize were caused by milk proteins."*
>
> **Dr. John McDougall**

This does not mean that we do not need calcium in the diet. We do. There are sources of calcium which do not create the problems dairy products do. Green vegetables, such as broccoli, collard greens, and kale, are loaded with calcium. Fortified orange juice and many common varieties of beans are also rich in calcium. The key is to insure that these foods are included in the diet, while also reducing the loss of calcium from the body by limiting protein intake to reasonable amounts.

Sexual Functioning

Not long ago, I was giving a lecture in Lubbock, Texas. As I spelled out the evidence on how a bad diet leads to heart disease and strokes, a group of students in the back of the room began to mutter and complain. They were studying beef and pork production and were not about to hear criticisms of the agriculture industry. I described the process of atherosclerosis, commonly known as "hardening of the arteries," which chokes off the blood supply to the heart muscle, causing heart attacks and often death. The same process occurs in the arteries to the brain, leading to strokes—the death of a portion of the brain. Howls of laughter came from the back of the room, sprinkled with heckling. They did not want to believe the message.

"You can laugh all you want," I said. "But this process of atherosclerosis doesn't just cause heart attacks. It also causes *impotence*." Total silence fell on the room. Suddenly, we were not discussing the remote afflictions of middle age. The very essence of masculinity was threatened.

Can diet be related to impotence? The answer is yes. A study of 440 impotent men was published in the *Lancet* in January, 1985.[11]

The risk factors that have been identified for heart disease were present in the impotent men far more commonly than in the general population (See Chapter 1). Just as a loss of blood flow to the heart muscle leads to the death of a portion of the heart, the loss of blood flow to the genitals interferes with sexual potency. Ultimately, impotence can result. The study concluded that "the increase in the frequency of impotence with age is mainly related to arteriosclerotic changes . . . ." The high-fat, high-cholesterol diet is a principal culprit.

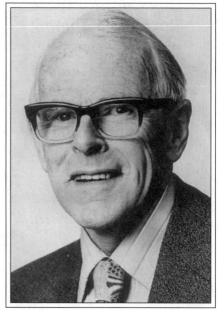

Dr. Denis Burkitt

But the connections between diet and impotence do not end there. As we noted in this chapter, diet contributes to diabetes. In turn, diabetes often leads to impotence, both because atherosclerosis is more aggressive in diabetics and because gradual damage to peripheral nerves also occurs in many diabetics. Above, we reviewed some basics of the dietary control of diabetes.

Diet is also an important factor in hypertension, which also contributes to impotence by way of its effect on atherosclerosis. In addition, some of the medications used in the treatment of hypertension can interfere with sexual functioning. Methyldopa (Aldomet) frequently leads to impotence. Guanethidine commonly causes inhibition of ejaculation. Ironically, although high blood pressure can be a very serious condition, it often has no symptoms that the patient can feel. So when men are treated with drugs which cause impotence, they may find they have little motivation to take the drugs as prescribed. Because hypertension is a serious condition, however, any change in medications should be discussed with your doctor. In Chapter 1, we looked at how a high-fat diet can lead to high blood pressure and how a lower-fat diet, particularly a vegetarian diet, can lower blood pressure. Some people will continue to need medications, but many can use a dietary approach instead.

McDougall strongly encourages giving the dietary approach a try. "Many men on blood pressure pills are impotent," McDougall said. "I'll ask if they'd like to try beans and rice instead." In his years of practice in Hawaii, McDougall consistently noticed that Asian men on traditional diets which omitted dairy products and con-tained relatively little meat not only lived longer, they also remained sexually functional throughout their lives. "Sometimes men would start new families when they were 70 years old," McDougall said. "They could function sexually at 70 years old. And they were going to see their children grow up and go to high school and so on. They didn't plan on dying at 72. They planned to live to be 85 or 90, and so they did, and in good health."

Denis Burkitt on the Role of Medicine

In his pioneering research on cancer, and, more recently, on nutrition, Denis Burkitt's methods were as unique as his findings. Burkitt solved his medical questions, not with test tubes and laboratory equipment mainly, but by carefully studying popula-tions. For the most part, the information he needed was not readily available. So he went out and got it. He spent a tremendous amount of time traveling around Africa and much of the rest of the world, including places beyond the reach of roads, to see the places which were struck by disease and those which were not. Then he analyzed his data to see what he could find.

Initially, he discovered, and cured, Burkitt's lymphoma. He then took on a much bigger target in trying to reform the dietary habits of Western countries. But he also recognized the need to redirect medical research and practice.

"First of all, medical students ought to have in their curriculum a course on nutrition and not waste their time learning about cancer surgery or heart surgery until later in their specialist careers," Burkitt said.

"When I worked for twelve years at the Medical Research Council, my senior used to adjudicate all applications for grants. He wrote two words at the end of every request: 'So what?' Now if all research grants had 'So what?' written at the end of them, you'd cut them down by about three-quarters. An awful lot of them have no practical application. And in this stage of life, we ought to be looking for practical applications."

Is Burkitt suggesting that much of the research going on nowadays isn't really worth a whole lot? "Absolute waste of money. And there is one other thing. The National Cancer Institute asked me to lecture there. I started my lecture by saying I thought the biggest defect in cancer research today was specializing in cancer, which must have shaken them a bit. If you try to find out the cause of a disease like bowel cancer, you've got to look at all the other diseases associated with it. You see, I get credited for the idea that fiber might be protective against bowel cancer, but I got into that by recognizing that you never get diverticular disease in a community that hasn't got a high rate of bowel cancer.* They go together. Now, you forget about the cancer; you look at the diverticular disease, and you find that diverticular disease is related to low-fiber diets. Couldn't cancer be the same? But the cancer specialist seldom looks at anything except cancer. He doesn't even record polyps in his registry. And since colon cancer is nearly always derived from polyps in America, and there are a hundred or a thousand times as many polyps as cancers, why not get rid of cancer research altogether and look for the cause of polyps? Then you've got the answer.

"I was in Cincinnati some years ago, and after my lecture a man came to speak to me. He told me that he was chosen by the government to advise people on diet and health. He said, 'I understand what you're talking about, but I'm not going to advise anybody until I understand all the mechanisms and have double-blind trials, and what have you.' 'Well,' I said, 'Diverticular disease is going to take a sixty-year trial, so it'll be your grandson writing up the last paper. If you were on a pier and your son fell into the water, I know what you'd do. If you had a life jacket in your hand, you wouldn't throw it to him. You'd say, "I'm not quite sure of the specific gravity of this life jacket, and I don't really know whether it fits my son. I think I'll go back to the lab. I'll do three more weeks' work on my life jacket, then I'll come back to the harbor and, if Jimmy's still swimming around, I'll throw him the life jacket" But we don't work that way. This is armchair science.

"Fiber is something which we didn't understand, didn't know how to measure, and didn't know what it did until less than twenty years ago. So we said, 'Let's take it out.' We didn't understand tonsils until we discovered T-cells and B-cells in the early 1960s. What did we do with tonsils? Took them out. We didn't understand the appendix—chop it out. There have been several papers now showing that if you have had your tonsils and your appendix out, you've got a bigger chance of getting certain cancers, notably Hodgkins' Disease, than if you keep them. We didn't understand hemorrhoids—nip 'em off. But this is the kind of arrogant approach to medicine: if you don't understand something, you cut it out. And now we recognize that you can't do that. God didn't give us any of these things just for fun."

Diverticulosis is a condition in which pouches form in the wall of the large intestine (colon). When these pouches become inflamed, the condition is known as diverticulitis.

Chapter 6

Foods and the Mind

"One cannot think well, love well, sleep well,
if one has not dined well."

Virginia Woolf

Foods affect the brain in many ways. Some foods make us sleep. Others help us stay alert. Sugar can have either positive or negative effects, depending on what else is part of the meal. Alcohol, likewise, can be a sedative or a stimulant, depending on timing and genetics. Even NutraSweet can affect brain chemistry. Foods can affect a child's performance in school and even the basic functioning of the child's brain.

Alcohol

Alcohol is a universal sedative. Under its influence, anxieties melt away and inhibitions dissolve. We find ourselves talking, laughing, singing, or doing other things we would normally do with more restraint.

Alcohol's Dr. Jekyll and Acetaldehyde

Some of alcohol's effects are not due to the alcohol itself, but to its first cousin, *acetaldehyde*. This compound is naturally produced from alcohol as the alcohol molecule is broken down in the body. Acetaldehyde is, in turn, broken down and excreted. But if acetaldehyde is made from alcohol faster than it can be removed, it builds up in the blood stream. Unlike alcohol, whose effects are usually experienced as pleasant, acetaldehyde may cause very unpleasant effects. If acetaldehyde builds up, it causes a flushed appearance, headache, nausea and vomiting, rapid pulse, and low blood pressure.

A glass of wine or other alcohol promotes sleep. But acetaldehyde is stimulating and may cause early morning awakening. For some people, particularly women, rather little acetaldehyde accumulates; for others, the amounts are quite significant. So while alcohol may promote sleep, one might find oneself wide awake before dawn, unable to return to sleep.

Aspartame: Brain Effects of NutraSweet®

NutraSweet has taken the diet food industry by storm. Research shows, however, that the chemical sweetener may be inadvertently causing a storm of a different sort: a storm inside our brain cells. Aspartame, the chemical marketed as NutraSweet, is a combination of two amino acids—phenylalanine and aspartic acid. Richard Wurtman, M.D., a researcher at the Massachusetts Institute of Technology in Cambridge, Massachusetts, found that the chemical may promote convulsions. He published in the medical journal, *The Lancet*, reports of three people who had had grand mal seizures, collapsing as their muscles jerked violently, after consuming large amounts of NutraSweet-flavored soft drinks.[1]

Wurtman had been hired as a consultant to G.D. Searle and Co., NutraSweet's manufacturer. But while working with Searle, Wurtman found and reported on the seizure cases. These people had never had seizures before. There was no reason why they should have had seizures, except for the effect Wurtman suspected NutraSweet had on their brain cells. The company did not listen to Wurtman's concerns. He came to believe that Searle was not particularly interested in what he had to say.

Wurtman believed the company was not honestly dealing with the safety issue. "I still trust them as far as I can throw your building," he wrote to Sanford A. Miller, of the Food and Drug Administration. As the case reports of seizures accumulated, Wurtman became more and more concerned about the connection between NutraSweet and seizures.

"We now have over 200 cases of previously healthy young adults who had a full grand mal seizure associated with consuming, over a period of time, large amounts of aspartame."

Dr. Richard Wurtman

"I thought this was more than a chance coincidence," Wurtman said, "because there are good reasons why aspartame might be expected to make people more likely to have seizures. It contains phenylalanine. When you consume aspartame, something happens to your blood and your brain that never previously happened in man's evolutionary history. It was only after somebody invented a food like aspartame that it was possible to do the experiment asking, when you raise phenylalanine in the brain, what happens? It's an experiment that I think I would rather not have seen done. Because, of all the amino acids, phenylalanine is the one for which there is the best evidence of neurotoxicity."

Phenylalanine can damage brain cells. High levels of phenylalanine develop in children with a disease called phenylketonuria, or PKU. Profound brain damage is often the result. When we consume aspartame, we are essentially drinking phenylalanine. How much NutraSweet can we consume and still be sure that the phenylalanine levels in the brain are safe? No one knows. Wurtman advises pregnant women and small children to stay off aspartame completely. Phenylalanine affects brain cells directly and interferes with substances in the brain which are responsible for preventing seizures.

"We now have over 200 cases of previously healthy young adults who had a full grand mal seizure associated with consuming, over a period of time, large amounts of aspartame," Wurtman said. "Many of these people first have headaches, deja vu, or other symptoms before seizures begin."

Canadian researchers studied children who had had seizures previously, unrelated to aspartame. They found that the chemical made their brain wave patterns even more abnormal, suggesting that it might make existing seizures worse.[2]

At Children's Hospital in Washington, D.C., Dr. C. Keith Conners conducted sophisticated studies on how various nutrients affect children. Conners has found that NutraSweet can cause a variety of physical complaints: headaches, nausea, lethargy, diarrhea, and stomach aches. But it can also produce behavioral effects. One four-year-old had a particularly serious reaction.

"The boy exhibited a profound hyperactivity that came on very suddenly. He became overactive for 36 to 48 hours and didn't sleep, hardly ate, became agitated and quite wild, and had to be restrained. He ran full-tilt into the wall, repeatedly knocking himself down. He became so agitated. This happened on several occasions. Even after he was restricted from all aspartame-containing foods, when he inadvertently received some, the episodes were repeated." If he had Kool-Aid sweetened with sugar there was no problem. But Kool-Aid with NutraSweet caused the bizarre symptoms to recur.

The problems don't end there. "It's turning out that if you open a can of diet soda," Dr. Wurtman said, "you find in that can a lot more than just the aspartame you put in. The chemical is very unstable.

By the time you open the can, five to ten percent of it has rearranged to an entirely different chemical called beta-aspartame. Does it enter the brain? I don't know. No one's ever studied it. Now there are seven compounds that people are aware of that are present in the can of soda to which aspartame had been added."

Unfortunately, the marketing of aspartame has been full speed ahead, and industry has had little interest in the consequences. "They're just very flagrantly dishonest," Wurtman said. "They lead the listener to believe that phenylalanine is phenylalanine, whether you get it in protein or you get it in aspartame, and that simply isn't true."

> *"It's turning out that if you open a can of diet soda, you find a lot more than just the aspartame you put in. Five to ten percent of it has rearranged to an entirely different chemical.*
>
> **Dr. Richard Wurtman**

Many other researchers have begun to look at the effects of aspartame, and have found mixed results. Many have concluded that it is safe.[3] On the other hand, it is now apparent that supplementing individual amino acids can be dangerous. In the body, aspartame breaks down chemically to its two amino acids, plus a bit of methanol. It is safe to say that no one needs any of these as dietary supplements.

How You Eat Affects How You Sleep

A good night's sleep cures a myriad of ills. In dreams we turn over the troubles of the previous day and put them aside. Our muscles rest, and our body chemistry completes its many nocturnal tasks. When we sleep well, we are ready to take on the next day. When sleep is disrupted, though, we are irritable and easily fatigued. Physical and emotional pains hurt more.

Many people report that dietary habits affect their sleep. For example, large meals late in the evening sometimes interfere with sleep. A lighter dinner earlier in the evening may help. In addition, we can manipulate the brain's chemistry to promote a good night's sleep. *Serotonin* is a natural chemical in the brain. Among many other functions, serotonin acts as a hypnotic. When serotonin is more plentiful, we feel sleepy. The concentration of serotonin in the brain depends on the balance of proteins and carbohydrates in the foods we eat.

Pure carbohydrate meals increase serotonin. Carbohydrates are sugars or combinations of sugars. A piece of cake or pie or a glass of juice before bed increases the amount of serotonin in the brain and helps us sleep. The sandman would be more effective if he would leave his sand at home and distribute jelly donuts instead.

But this effect is blocked by protein. If there is much protein in the foods we have eaten, serotonin levels will not rise, and the sedative effect will not occur. So to feel sleepy, have a high-carbohydrate snack, such as fruit juice or cake. To avoid drowsiness after meals, have a mixture of carbohydrate and protein.

In the morning, we want to feel alert. So we will block the carbohydrate effect with a small amount of protein. A mixture of

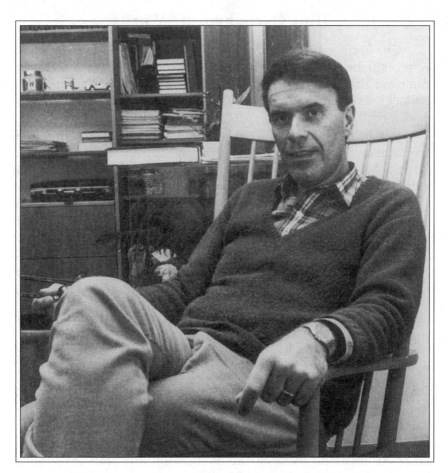

Dr. Richard Wurtman

protein and carbohydrate has none of the serotonin-enhancing effect of pure carbohydrate. Very little protein is needed to block the carbohydrate effect. If protein makes up about ten percent of the meal, the effect is blocked.[4] Happily, most foods contain both protein and carbohydrate. Oatmeal, for example, contains both, as do other breakfast cereals and whole wheat toast. These foods contain enough protein to block the serotonin effect.

The usual American breakfast has a large amount of protein in eggs, bacon, and sausage, but these foods have an enormous content of fat and cholesterol. In Mexico and parts of England, a breakfast may consist of beans on toast. While it sounds odd to Americans, this breakfast is a way of combining protein (far more than is needed to block the carbohydrate effect) with carbohydrate, while eliminating the unwanted fat and cholesterol.

How Carbohydrate Works

The brain makes many of the chemicals it needs from proeins. A protein molecule is like a string of beads. When we digest proteins, the "beads" come off, each bead being an amino acid molecule. It is these amino acids that are used to build what the body needs.

The brain makes serotonin from a particular amino acid called tryptophan. The more tryptophan that passes from the blood stream into the brain, the more serotonin it makes. But the brain does not automatically get as much tryptophan as it can use. Only so many amino acid molecules can pass from the blood stream into the brain at a time. Tryptophan is competing with the other amino acids to get into the brain.

Here is where carbohydrate works. Carbohydrate stimulates the release of insulin, which ushers many of the competing amino acids out of the blood stream. (Insulin also does the same to sugar.) Tryptophan is left behind because it is attached to a carrier molecule which prevents it from leaving the blood. Now it has less competition for getting into the brain, where it can produce serotonin.

It is a complicated path, but it works: carbohydrate increases insulin, which increases the amount of tryptophan that gets to the brain, which increases serotonin, which makes us fall asleep. Studies have shown that the same regimen can raise the pain threshold, so that hurts hurt a little less. [5,6]

Dr. Wurtman had originally thought that protein would increase tryptophan levels in the brain. After all, protein contains tryptophan as one of its amino acid building blocks. But he found that protein did not increase the amount of tryptophan getting to the brain. Sometimes, in fact, it actually reduced it. "It took us a while before we acknowledged it," Wurtman said, "because the experiments didn't work the way we expected them to. And the reason is this: Protein contains some tryptophan. But it contains a much larger amount of the other amino acids that compete with tryptophan." There is just too much competition. There are no foods that supply tryp-tophan without an overly generous supply of its competitors.

"There was an article in the *New York Times* saying that if you want to feel sleepy, eat tryptophan, and the way to do that is by having turkey," Wurtman said. "I sent them a letter and they published a correction. There is no protein source that will raise brain tryptophan. All natural proteins contain so little tryptophan compared with the other amino acids that they have either no effect or they lower brain tryptophan.

"You have to eat carbohydrate. You can use carbohydrate like a drug, up to a point. You can decide that for a few hours you would like to increase your brain serotonin, because you want to go to sleep, or because you feel jittery or what have you. I know a number of people who do quite well having a piece of cake and some orange juice at bedtime. It has a very nice effect."

Food and Your Mood

Some people have what may be a natural deficiency of serotonin. They are often depressed, particularly in the winter months when there is less daylight. This annual cycle of depression is termed Seasonal Affective Disorder (SAD). Many people with SAD crave carbohydrates, perhaps as a natural way to increase serotonin in the brain. The carbohydrates need not be sweet. Starchy carbohydrates are craved as well and raise serotonin just as effectively.

A research study at the Massachusetts Institute of Technology compared two groups of overweight people: "carbohydrate cravers" and those who do not have this tendency. After a meal of pure carbohydrates, those who were not carbohydrate cravers often felt worse. It made them sleepy or irritable. But the carbohydrate cravers had a very different reaction to the pure carbohydrate meals.

"It did not make them sleepy or grumpy," Wurtman said. "It actually improved their mood significantly. It's tempting to specu-

late that carbohydrate cravers, perhaps, don't have enough serotonin for whatever reason."

The carbohydrate-seeking behavior appears to be a way to
restore serotonin balance. So carbohydrate cravers feel better after
a carbohydrate meal. Others, however, feel worse, unless the carbohydrate is mixed with proteins.

Sugar and Children

For children, sugar does more than cause cavities. It clearly
affects the way the brain works. Sometimes sugar makes children
inattentive and diminishes their ability to think and react. Under
certain circumstances, however, sugar actually helps brain function. The key is in what else the child has eaten.

At Children's Hospital in Washington D. C., Conners tested the
effects of sugar on children. If children had had a mainly carbohydrate breakfast, such as plain white toast, a sugar snack later in the
day would impair their attention span and slow their reaction time.
But if the breakfast contained more protein, sugar actually improved
mental functioning. The carbohydrate breakfast probably led to an
increase in serotonin levels in the brain. Sugar aggravated this
effect. But adding protein to the breakfast could block the effect.

The amount of sugar Conners used in the study was consider-
able—about the amount combined in a large piece of cherry pie and
a chocolate candy bar. This is a sizable quantity, but not out of the
range of many children's eating habits.

Conners showed that the effects of sugar could even be seen in
brain waves measured on the electroencephalogram (EEG). "In one
of the tests we had electrodes attached to the scalp so we could
measure the brain response," he said. "We know that the brain is
normally asymmetrical and that the two hemispheres of the brain
function quite differently. Verbal functions, on the whole, are on
one side of the brain and spatial functions are on the other side. In
this case, the asymmetry that is normally there was abolished by the
carbohydrate. It was as though one side of the brain had been
compromised by this temporary load.

"Sugar has its largest effect within an hour," Conners said, "but
the effects continue throughout the morning. A child whose reaction was slowed gets even slower during the later part of the day,
even though the blood sugar has returned to normal." But the effect
was totally offset by having protein at breakfast. With protein and
sugar together, the children Conners studied did very well.

What about fruit sugars, that is, the fructose in fruit and in
honey? Conners found fructose no better than table sugar. "We

compared fructose with sucrose (table sugar) and didn't really see any notable behavioral differences," Conners said. "In the lay literature, fructose is seen to be the 'good sugar,' particularly in the form of honey, and sucrose is the 'bad sugar.' In fact, you're probably doing more harm to yourself by eating honey from all the junk which is cooked in with it than you are by eating pure table sugar."

Children need breakfasts which combine carbohydrate and protein. Oatmeal or wheat cereals, for example, naturally combine both protein and carbohydrate.

Hyperactivity and the Feingold Diet

Hyperactive children are often restless and fidgety. They may run and climb at a pace that would exhaust other children. They may do poorly in school, which is often wrongly attributed to misbehavior.

The current diagnostic term for this syndrome is Attention Deficit Disorder, because one of the most common findings is an inability to focus attention for more than a brief period. Learning disabilities are also common in these children. Subtle abnormalities of the brain are probably responsible for the hyperactivity and the learning troubles these children experience.

In the 1970s, Dr. Ben Feingold popularized a dietary treatment for hyperactivity. Feingold, a pediatric allergist, noticed that the increasing incidence of hyperactivity in America paralleled the increasing use of artificial flavors and colors in foods. He hypothesized that hyperactivity was caused by a sensitivity to these additives and devised a diet that eliminated them. In addition, because some people who are allergic to food dyes are also sensitive to aspirin and related compounds, called salicylates, he also eliminated salicylate-containing foods, such as tomatoes, cucumbers, and fruits. With his diet, Feingold found dramatic improvements in the behavior of hyperactive children. As many as two-thirds of hyperactive children improved.

Feingold published his findings in *Why Your Child is Hyperactive* (Random House, 1985). As his interest in hyperactivity developed, one of the researchers whose works he read was Keith Conners. In turn, Conners tested Feingold's hypothesis.

At first, it appeared that Feingold was right. Conners confirmed that about two-thirds of children seemed to improve on the diet. But Conners became concerned that it was not the diet that was helping, but rather the parents' expectation that the children should improve. So he did another study, using hidden food additives. He gave children two kinds of cookies. Some contained food dye. Others were placebo cookies with no food dye.

"The mother of the very first patient called up the next day after receiving the cookie and said, 'I don't know what you put in that cookie, but whatever it is, I'm taking the kid out of the study, because he has gone berserk. He took a hammer and went next door and beat up the neighbor's motorcycle, he cut up our couch and just went wild. So those food dyes you put in that cookie are driving him crazy, and I'm taking him out of the study.' Well, as luck would have it, that child received placebo cookies the first day. He was responding to his own expectations of what ought to be happening when he eats a bad thing."

So is the Feingold diet just a placebo? "If you just put everybody on the diet, absolutely two-thirds of them get remarkably better," Conners said. "As soon as you do it in a double-blind fashion, those effects disappear. So it really means that if a person believes in the treatment, they will get better. It's largely a placebo effect. Feingold was misled by these rather dramatic changes into thinking they were real because he didn't believe that placebos could be that effective. Placebos are very powerful. When they're not controlled, they mislead even the best scientific observers. Dr. Feingold was a true humanist and a very genuine and committed man, but he essentially dropped his scientific guard at the wrong time."

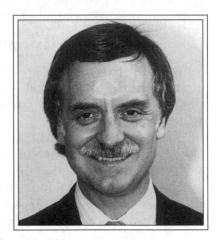

Dr. C. Keith Conners

That does not mean that the Feingold diet is totally ineffective. There does seem to be a small group of children who do, in fact, respond well to the diet. "In almost all the studies there have been one or two kids where there seems to be a pretty regular effect," Conners said. "We found when we started using more sensitive measures that there were a few such kids, usually younger kids."

Conners urges, though, that medical problems and the Feingold diet not be used as reasons to avoid looking at problems in the family that may be contributing to a child's difficulties. "Diets may be used as an argument against changing your own behavior and against examining family process problems that are more subtle and perhaps important." Foods are a part of the puzzle of hyperactivity, taking their place along with other pieces that are also important.

Alzheimer's Disease

One and one-half to two million Americans have Alzheimer's disease. Its main characteristic is dementia, that is, the loss of intellectual capacities. For some, the illness occurs early, between about 40 and 60 years of age. For others, the disease occurs only late in life.

The search for causes has turned up some interesting leads. People with Alzheimer's disease have been found to have aluminum in their brains. Autopsies showed that aluminum concentrates in the parts of the brain most affected by the disease. Is aluminum the cause? No one knows. Perhaps aluminum has nothing to do with causing the disease and was simply drawn to the damaged parts of the brain. But it may well be that aluminum actually does the damage.

"Unfortunately, we still don't know the answer," Wurtman said. "We do have more reason to worry now, I think. In the last few years very compelling data have been adduced showing a clear relationship between aluminum silicate and the two cardinal lesions of Alzheimer's disease, namely the plaques and tangles in the brain." Plaques and neurofibrillary tangles are microscopic abnormalities found in the brains of patients with Alzheimer's disease.

"If you analyze brain samples from people who have died of Alzheimer's disease, there's a very tight association between aluminum and the neurofibrillary tangles. A group of investigators recently found the same thing with plaques. So the question is, is it that the sick cell somehow attracts and binds aluminum? Or is aluminum somehow involved in causing the sickness? And here I don't think one knows the answer."

Until we know more we should be careful about aluminum. The main sources of aluminum are certain antacids, aluminum cans and cookware, and some processed cheeses. It is certainly easy to live without each of these. There is also a small amount of aluminum in common table salt and other packaged foods.

There is also evidence that people with Alzheimer's disease have too little of a neurotransmitter chemical, *acetylcholine*, in the brain. Research studies have looked at ways of stimulating acetylcholine production through diet. These have relied on giving nutrients called *choline* and *phosphatidylcholine* (also called *lecithin*), which the brain turns into acetylcholine. Some investigators have suggested that if lecithin is given long enough, it may slow or stop the progression of the disease for some patients, particularly older patients.

These supplements may work by stopping the destruction of brain cells. Brain cells that are hungry for acetylcholine may actually take choline from their own cell membranes in order to make it, a process referred to as "autocannibalism." "It may be that autocannibalism is part of the process of Alzheimer's disease," Wurtman said. "When you give people supplemental choline, then they stop breaking down their own membranes. Some might get a little bit better too, either because you've saved some sick membranes or because you have increased acetylcholine release from them."

> *"In the last few years very compelling data have been adduced showing a clear relationship between aluminum silicate and the two cardinal lesions of Alzheimer's disease."*
>
> **Dr. Richard Wurtman**

Where do we find choline in the diet? "You find very little free choline," Wurtman said, "except in a few vegetables like cauliflower, which is rich in choline. But most of the choline you find in the diet is in the form of phosphatidylcholine or lecithin, which is present in eggs and glandular meats, like liver. It's present in soybeans. It's used as an emulsifying agent in chocolate."

Eggs and organ meats are very high in cholesterol, and should be avoided. It would certainly be unwise to try to counteract Alzheimer's disease with foods that may promote a stroke or heart attack. Cauliflower is safe on both counts. But purified lecithin is what current research relies on. Researchers on Alzheimer's disease use doses of lecithin that are far higher than those available in foods.

"I hasten to add that one should not run off to the health food store and buy lecithin there," Wurtman said. "Even if it's called pure lecithin, by a quirk in the labeling laws, it will contain perhaps only 20 percent lecithin or less. But now several companies are making purified lecithin in the form of capsules or food-based preparations available to psychiatrists.

"Most people probably consume on the order of maybe 200 to 400 milligrams of choline per day. The doses of lecithin that are used in the study of Alzheimer's disease probably supply two to three grams of choline per day. By taking a large amount of purified lecithin, you're going to have an effect on brain acetylcholine, and ameliorate some conditions which seem to be related to increased acetylcholine."

The Mind's Eye on the Dinner Plate

Why should nature have allowed the brain to be battered about by something as trivial as our last meal? Why should carbohydrates and proteins be able to change neurotransmitter levels in the brain? It appears that this is the brain's way of monitoring our dietary intake. The brain tells us when to start or stop eating and what kinds of foods to select, often with great specificity. Neurotransmitters play a part in this regulatory process and change depending on what we are eating.

"If you were to count up all the foods you eat per week," Wurtman said, "and determine what percentage of the calories come from protein or carbohydrate, you'd find remarkable stability. And you are totally unaware of that. Well, your brain isn't. You think you are eating because the food smells good or because it's time to eat. To some extent you are. But in reality, your brain is choosing nutrients.

"I think that this mechanism was chosen by evolution in order, for instance, to keep the bear from only eating honey. Certain things taste very good, and that's dangerous. If the bear just ate honey, he wouldn't be a healthy bear."

Unfortunately, although our brain carefully balances our selections of carbohydrate and protein, it does not protect us from eating things that are unhealthy. The biggest problem seems to be the amount of fat we consume. Nearly half our calories each day come from fat. We choose fatty hamburgers, fried chicken, french fries, and other greasy foods. These selections, never vetoed by the brain, lead to heart disease, cancer, an epidemic of obesity, and numerous other problems. Although people have searched for connections between fatty foods and the brain from many years (Sir Andrew in Shakespear's *Twelfth Night* said, "I am a great eater of beef and I believe it does harm to my wit."), these relationships are not yet elucidated. There does not seem to be a neurochemical that is

> *"You think you are eating because the food smells good, or because it's time to eat. But in reality, your brain is choosing nutrients. I think that this mechanism was chosen by evolution in order to keep the bear from only eating honey."*
> **Dr. Richard Wurtman**

automatically affected by fat in the diet. So, unfortunately, fat comes along for the ride. If our brain is seeking out carbohydrate and chooses ice cream, then a lot of fat will be part of the meal. If on the other hand, it chooses rice as the source of carbohydrate, very little fat will be consumed. "Through our evolution this was not much of a problem," Wurtman said, "because fat was always very expensive. People did not have the capacity, unless they killed a walrus or something, of having enormous amounts of fat. But now fat is so cheap and available that we find large amounts of it present with the carbohydrates and proteins that we eat. And I really think that's the problem."

Fat is often craved in its many forms. At a previous time in our evolution, this made sense. Fat is a calorie-dense food. A gram of fat has more than twice the calories (nine) of a gram of carbohydrate or protein (four). By taking advantage of fatty foods on those rare occasions when they were available, our ancestors found a rich source of calories. But now that is the last thing we need.

Remembering Our Dietary Past

Prior to a century or two ago, the production of foods was a very different process than it is today. Flours were largely unrefined. Refined sugars were less available. Aluminum-containing antacids were not on our shelves. NutraSweet was not something we thought we needed.

Dietary traditions have often been ritualized in cultural practices. In the Jain culture in India, for example, food is not consumed after dark. While this is for several reasons, it is likely to minimize the disruption of sleep that may occur after a large meal.

Conners said, "In most religions, at what I would call their highest level, the level of the inner circle of practitioners, the same proscriptions about diet have obtained. Whether you're Moslem, Jewish, Buddhist, or Mormon, they all preach moderation and using food in a very skillful way to augment your main life goal. They also tend, on the whole, to dislike killing and to have proscriptions against animal food."

There is some value to recalling the past. For most of our history, animal foods were a smaller part of the diet. Strokes and heart disease were correspondingly less common. Without refining, foods contained a helpful balance of nutrients. The effect on amino acid levels, and therefore on neurotransmitters, was likely to have been more balanced. Our fragile brain cells were less often assaulted by unfamiliar chemicals and better protected when assaults occurred.

Chapter 7

Clues to the Natural Human Diet

The clear waters of Lake Tanganyika reach to the shores of Gombe, a strip of rugged, beautiful country in the Kigoma region of Tanzania. It was here in Gombe that Jane Goodall came in July, 1960, to study chimpanzees at the suggestion of paleoanthropologist Louis Leakey. Her studies of chimpanzees and what they eat tell us much about the natural diet of the human animal. There is also human evidence of our dietary development, as we will learn from Leakey's famous son, Richard. But first, let's take a brief look at our primate relatives.

For some time after Dr. Goodall's arrival, the chimpanzees cautiously avoided her approach. She had to observe at a distance through binoculars. But gradually the chimpanzees discovered there was nothing to fear and accepted the human tag-along. Eventually she took on field assistants and students who helped with observations and reporting in what was to become the longest continuous field study of any living creature. In the process, she has come to know the chimpanzees as individuals. Each has a unique life story Goodall has been able to observe. Chimps have been born. Others have died. Affection and playfulness, power struggles, and keen awareness of social structure are ingrained in chimpanzee life.

Fruits, Seeds, and Medicinal Plants

What is the natural diet of primates? Spam and roast beef sandwiches? Frozen yogurt? Kidney pie? If we can judge from the chimpanzees, it is mostly fruit.

Fruits typically make up more than half of the chimps' diet. Goodall's notes contain vivid descriptions, such as Passion, the careless chimp who did not bother to wipe off the mess of sticky juice from the strychnos fruits she had been eating, while seated next to her, her three-year-old son, Pax, meticulously wiped his chin clean with blades of grass.

"The chimps spend a great deal of time eating the fruit that is in season," Goodall said. "Probably the most significant is the fruit of the oil nut palm, because the trees have their own individual cycles. The fruit clusters ripen one after the other throughout the year, so the chimps can get palm nuts in virtually any month."

Just as human civilizations develop their culturally favorite foods, chimps do the same. These traditions are passed from parent to child in each succeeding generation.

"The oil nut palm is the most dramatic example," Goodall said. "The Gombe chimps eat the fruit; they eat the pith; they eat the dried male flower cluster—at least they chew and spit out the fiber; and they also eat the dead wood from the trunk. At Mahale, by contrast, chimps don't eat any part of this palm. In the Tai Forest of the Ivory Coast the chimps have not been seen eating the palm nuts. They do, however, commonly eat the pith. In Liberia, they crack open the hard kernels using stone hammers and eat the nuts inside; these are not eaten at Gombe or at Tai.

"There are differences in methods of feeding as well. The chimps at Gombe eat the strychnos fruit by cracking it open against a stone, and the Mahale chimps break open the fruit with their teeth. So there are very clear cultural differences between different populations.

"I suspect that new cultural traditions of this sort are mostly started by infants," Goodall said, "because infants are the ones who are always exploring, testing, trying. Sometimes an adult will

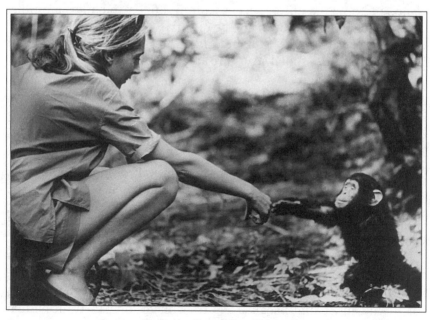

Dr. Jane Goodall and friend

actually prevent an infant from feeding on a fruit that is not a part of the adult diet, even though we know it not to be poisonous. When I offered new foods to infants, they were usually interested, but sometimes others prevented them from actually eating them. An elder sister flicked biscuit crumbs away from her infant brother, a mother seized a piece of pa-paya from her child, sniffed it, then hurled it away, and so on."

After fruits, leaves are the next largest part of the diet, comprising 10 to 40 percent of the chimpanzee menu, followed by seeds and blossoms. The chimps have even found a medicinal leaf, the aspilia leaf. "There is evidently an antibiotic in these leaves,"Goodall said. "Instead of chewing them, the chimp sort of rubs them against the roof of his mouth with his tongue, then swallows them whole."

The aspilia leaves have been shown to contain a natural chemical that helps prevent infections. Many human cultures have also made use of the aspilia leaves in medicines. The chimps may have made similar discoveries in wood and bark. They chew the fibers to extract the juices. Is it simply recreation, or is there some natural kind of medicine in the plant fibers? Few of the extracts have been analyzed, and, unlike humans, chimpanzees have no distinction between foods and medicines. "Perhaps some of the foods the chimps eat would be quite beneficial to humans," Goodall said, "from a nutritional as well as medical point of view."

On their diet of fruits and vegetation, the chimps remain amazingly healthy, free of most of the diseases that plague humans.

The Search for Clues to Our Past

There is little doubt that the wide travels which have taken our kind to every part of the globe began in Africa. North of Gombe, in neighboring Kenya, Richard Leakey searches for clues to the changing anatomy and behavior of our ancestors of millions of years ago. While the trail of bones and other remnants which could have told the story of our past was largely devoured in time like the bread crumbs of Hansel and Gretel, a few vital clues remain. In 1967, while flying along the eastern shore of Lake Turkana, Leakey noticed eroded layers of lake deposits which he judged would hold fossils of millions of years ago. He was right. The bones and stone tools that were the remnants of our human ancestors were buried under layer after layer of silt. Erosion has begun to uncover these long-buried clues from the past. The fossil specimens his team has found have been carefully examined. Bones have been analyzed by visual inspection, microscopic examination of surface scratch marks, and other techniques to reveal how humans evolved in the changing environment.

Can we say what made up the diet of early humans? Would our diet have been like that of a chimpanzee, relying on fruits, leaves, seeds, and other vegetation? "The diet of a primate such as a baboon or chimpanzee wouldn't be a bad pattern," Leakey said. "There's an awful lot of food available on the savannah that can be picked with the hands, from fruits, to tubers, to rhizomes, to plants above and below the ground, to insects. There was quite enough food on the African savannah in times of plenty for large primates to be very happy."

Are chimpanzees really a good model for the human diet? How close are we to chimpanzees in a biological sense? "Molecular biologists and geneticists have compared proteins and compared DNA and compared the whole spectrum of biochemical features," Leakey said. "They have established very convincingly that we are closer to the chimpanzee than a horse is to a donkey. We are extraordinarily similar."

> *"Molecular biologists and geneticists have established very convincingly that we are closer to the chimpanzee than a horse is to a donkey. We are extraordinarily similar."*
>
> **Dr. Richard Leakey**

But we are also very different. Baboons and chimpanzees have many anatomical differences from hominids, the name used for humans and our human-like predecessors. Chimpanzees have large canine teeth. Early humans, like modern humans, did not. As a result, if we ever caught an animal, tearing through its hide or cutting its flesh would have been an enormous struggle until the invention of stone tools much later. "You can't tear flesh by hand; you can't tear hide by hand," said Leakey. "Our anterior teeth are not suited for tearing flesh or hide. We don't have large canine teeth, and we wouldn't have been able to deal with food sources that required those large canines."

Until about two and a half million years ago, we had no stone tools. The sharp canine teeth some other primates use to occasionally kill and eat small mammals had been lost to our species by at least three and a half million years ago.

"It certainly is distinctive that the hominids don't have sharp, projective canines, and the non-hominids do," Leakey said. "When you go back to three or three and a half million years, there were some hominids with canines that were perhaps marginally larger than the modern human's, but it's not a significant difference. You've got to go further back to find the origin of that adaptation. The loss of projecting canines must relate to an adaptation of some kind. I don't think they'd just disappear."

Getting rid of large canine teeth allowed our ancestors to eat the available foods more easily. Vegetation was everywhere, and food processors and cooking equipment were not yet on the scene. So we ate a great deal of plants which were uncooked. Like cattle, horses, or other vegetarians, we needed molars for crushing food rather than knife-like incisors for cutting through flesh. Without the restriction of large canine teeth, our jaws were able to move somewhat side-to-side to crush vegetation.

"If you've got interlocking canines and third molars and you close your mouth, you're basically locking it anteriorly," Leakey said. "But if you've got smaller canines that don't lock anteriorly, you've got a far greater lateral movement. There could be some benefit from reducing the size of the canines and being able to chew foods differently."

Stone Tools and Scavenging

So presumably we were eating a diet that was more in line with the essentially vegetarian non-human primates on the savannah. Then, about two-and-a-half million years ago, crude stone tools made their first appearance. We still relied on fruits and other vegetation we could pick with our hands. But with stone tools we were able to cut apart a carcass if we got a hold of one. That, of course, was another matter. We were not quick like lions or tigers. Nor were we particularly strong. Our weapons were quite crude, and hunting was very inefficient. And why bother, anyway, in a land filled with fruits and lush vegetation? The beginning of meat-eating was probably not hunting at all. It was scavenging. In times of drought, when vegetation was scarce, we may have been forced to eat the left-overs of carnivores' prey.

"If you faced a narrowing of your dietary base because of environmental change of some kind—desiccation, whatever," Leakey said, "then the only way to maintain yourself would be to change your feeding strategy. One of the options seems to have been to increase the amount of meat. Now the only way to do that is to get

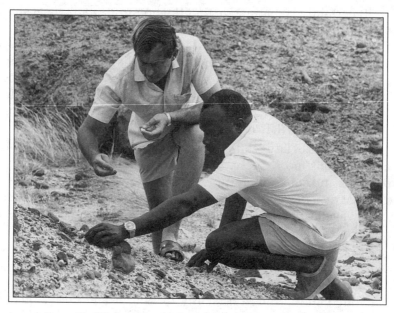

Dr. Richard Leakey and Mr. Kamoya Kimew

hold of it. If you're a bipedal primate and not particularly intelligent, the obvious way to do it is to scavenge. I mean, scavenging doesn't take a great deal of smarts. You've got to be fairly careful what you scavenge from, but in Africa on the savannah, there is invariably a lot of wasted meat on the remains. There is a wide range of scavengers: hyenas and jackals, birds, insects, and reptiles. It seems to me that a perfectly sensible new strategy is to scavenge for a while, taking from the remains of animals killed by more successful hunters—lions or other large carnivores."

Early humans, who would have had trouble catching and killing prey on their own, occasionally found left-overs waiting for them. "Lions never eat everything," Leakey said. "Lions leave anything from 10 percent to 80 percent of what they kill. Now there's quite a long line of different scavengers that have their own hierarchy, if you like, but a bipedal primate could quite easily move into that hierarchy without too much threat. I don't think that would have taken much to learn. But you're only going to be able to do that when you can cut the meat. The hyenas and vultures have got sharp equipment of their own, and you've got to be able to get at it yourself if you're going to compete with them."

The analysis of ancient animal bones supports the scavenging hypothesis. Patterns of scratches on these bones have revealed that stone tools were scraped over the bones after carnivorous teeth had cut into them, suggesting that the bones had been carnivores' prey which were then scraped clean by human scavengers.

The possibility of using stone tools to cut carcasses demanded degrees of reasoning and manipulation that had not previously occurred. It also demanded cultural changes as a new food source was exploited. "About two and a half million years ago, you suddenly find evidence of tools: sharp stones, stones that have been broken and have sharp edges," Leakey said. "These are invariably associated with bones of animals, suggesting meat in the diet in one form or another. That evidence coincides with the first appearance of an enlarged and modified brain shape. That process of cutting meat required a degree of mental equipment that was perhaps an advance over the primitive ancestral condition."

Some may imagine that early humans were essentially full-time hunters who ate nothing but meat. But the evidence does not support this idea. "Remember that the eating of meat on the African savannah," Leakey said, "although it's in big packages and you can share it, still accounts for a relatively small part of your diet. Even with the successful scavengers and successful hunters, meat is a rather small part of the diet, except in places like the Arctic, where in certain seasons meat is the only thing you can eat because there's nothing else to gather. But we are not carnivores and never have been carnivores, and that should be remembered. Some have become in modern times increasingly carnivorous because of the ready availability of meat from domestic animals. The excess of meat and the imbalance of the contemporary diet as a result of the domestication of cattle, sheep and goats, pigs, chickens, and fish, is, of course, something unusual."

"Forms of violence that so characterize contemporary times have absolutely no relationship to a hunting past. It reflects a total misunderstanding of the hunting urge, if there is such a thing as a hunting urge."

Dr. Richard Leakey

Hunting and Aggression

Cave paintings depict scenes of hunts. A history of hunting, real or imagined, might imply that earliest man had a certain amount of innate aggression that nowadays translates into wars and other forms of violence. Leakey disagrees. "A predator-prey relationship is a totally different thing from individual aggression where food is not its purpose. When you go off and kill a mammoth or kill a grasshopper, one is doing it because one's hungry. The urban violence, the interpersonal violence, the international violence, and other forms of violence that so characterize contemporary times have absolutely no relationship to a hunting past. It reflects a total misunderstanding of the hunting urge, if there is such a thing as a hunting urge."

Hunting in modern times, Leakey contends, has nothing to do with survival either. "That men, in particular, find great satisfaction in hunting and in showing their bravado has all to do with our hormones and our need to display. It is a male characteristic to display prowess in an area that attracts attention both from other males and presumably from breeding females. I think what we're seeing with these chaps who go off with great guns and shoot animals that really can't do them any harm is related to a breeding strategy, a sort of macho reproductive mating dance."

Evidence indicates that our species has thrived on a high-fiber diet of foods from plants. With little meat and no dairy products until relatively recently in the historical process, fat and cholesterol would have made a much more modest contribution to our diet than they do today. It has become more and more clear that a return to the diet of our past would be of great benefit. Just as medical research shows that meat-eating is responsible for an increase in risk of cancer, heart disease, and other illness, anthropological research has shown that our bodies were designed for an herbivorous menu. Adaptation to a new diet is a slow process. While we dine on twentieth century food, our bodies are made for quite a different diet indeed.

Chapter 8

Lessons from Around the World

In their search for an optimal diet, researchers have looked for groups of people who tend to stay healthy into advanced age. Of course, no country has a perfect diet or perfect health. But Asian countries do a much better job of holding cancer, heart disease, and many other serious conditions at arm's length than do Western countries.

China has provided, in a sense, a natural laboratory. Diets vary significantly from one part of the country to another, and people tend to stay in the same place all their lives, allowing relationships between diet and health to emerge.

Most nutrition researchers have ignored this opportunity. They have focused on single nutrients such as beta-carotene, vitamin C, fiber, or any one of the hundreds of others teased out of foods, and studied them in isolation. They study whether cigarette-smokers are healthier if they take a beta-carotene pill or whether meat-eaters do better with fiber supplements, consuming vast sums of money and yielding results that are often vague or conflicting.

T. Colin Campbell and his colleagues, Chen Junshi and Li Junyao of Beijing, China, and Richard Peto of Oxford University, tried a radically different approach. In one of the most ambitious nutrition research projects ever conducted, they exploited the natural dietary variations in China. They asked, not whether one or another vitamin supplement helps, but rather, what are the health effects that come from much more comprehensive differences in the diet.

Beginning in 1983, the team collected information about the typical foods of 65 Chinese provinces. They studied records of health and illness, and took blood samples and made other tests. In 1991, they published an 896-page monograph filled with their data, which they continue to analyze, along with the results of their subsequent and even larger studies. Their first findings were that, overall, Chinese diets are extraordinarily healthy by Western standards. Rice and other grains, vegetables, and legumes are consumed in much greater quantity than in the U.S. So while Americans get 37 percent of their calories from fat, the Chinese do far better. "Fat intake in China ranges from a low of 6% of calories to a high of 24%," Campbell said. "

And because the diet is plant-based, it avoids most of the ill effects that come from animal protein in Western diets. "Protein intake in China, on average, is about two-thirds of what it is in the West," Campbell said. "And the kind of protein that is consumed is very different. Only about 10% of the total protein intake is from animal sources, whereas here it is about 70%. As a percent of total calories, animal protein intake is about ten times higher here than in rural China."

The Power of a Plant-Based Diet

But even though their diets are better overall, there is a range of diets within China, which allows their effect on disease rates to be studied in detail.

The China Study suggests that a diet composed entirely of grains, vegetables, legumes, and fruits is superior to diets containing even small amounts of meat, poultry, or other animal products. "When only a small amount of animal products are added to the diet, up to 20% of total protein or so, it makes a significant difference," Campbell said. "When we compare people on diets that are virtually nil in animal protein with those for whom animal protein is upwards of twenty to thirty percent of the total protein intake, the cholesterol levels go from around 90 milligrams per deciliter to about 170 milligrams per deciliter. And these increases in cholesterol are associated with the emergence of the cancers and heart disease that are common in the West."

Recognition of the power of plant-based diets was quite a turnaround in Campbell's own life. "I was raised on a dairy farm," Campbell said. "I milked cows from the time I was five until I was twenty-one. We had our own garden and our own livestock for meat and dairy. When I went away to school, I eventually got my Ph.D. at Cornell in animal nutrition. I worked on a project to see how we might be able to produce animal protein more efficiently. So both my personal life as well as my professional life were entirely on the other end of the research findings that we've been getting."

Problems With Animal Protein

The China Study has highlighted particular risks from animal protein. Most people, of course, are more concerned about fat, because fat increases cholesterol and increases cancer risk. Should we be concerned about problems from too much protein?

"Definitely," Campbell said. "There is strong evidence in the scientific literature that when a reduction in fat is compared to a reduction in protein intake, the protein effect on blood cholesterol is more significant than the effect of saturated fat. Animal protein is a hypercholesterolemic agent. We can reduce cholesterol levels either by reducing animal protein intake or exchanging it for plant protein. Some of the plant proteins, particularly soy, have an impressive ability to reduce cholesterol. I really think that protein—both the kind and the amount—is more significant as far as cholesterol levels are concerned than is saturated fat, and certainly more significant than dietary cholesterol itself."

The reason for animal protein's dangerous effect on cholesterol is not entirely clear, but some clues have emerged. "We do know that the consumption of animal protein has a profound effect on enzymes that are involved in the metabolism of cholesterol and relatedchemicals," Campbell said. "This occurs very quickly—within hours after the consumption of the meal. "Whether it is the immune system, various enzyme systems, the uptake of carcinogens into the cells, or hormonal activities, animal protein generally only causes mischief. High fat intake still can be a problem, and we ought not to be consuming such high-fat diets. But I suggest that animal protein is more problematic in this whole diet/disease relationship than is total fat."

Of course, in the very recent past, animal protein was regarded as a healthful, if not essential, source of nutrition. The result is that Westerners tend to prefer to switch from one animal protein source to another, such as from beef to chicken breast, rather than to plant-based diets. Yet a switch from beef to poultry is not likely to help much, if at all. "The existing evidence suggests that this makes little or no sense," Campbell said. "It may reduce fat intake a bit, but even lean cuts of meat or poultry still contain around 20-40% of total

> *"Whether it is the immune system, various enzyme systems, the uptake of carcinogens into the cells, or hormonal activities, animal protein generally only causes mischief."*
>
> **Dr. T. Colin Campbell**

calories as fat, or even more. This is not going to get us very far. It might get our fat intake down a bit, but our protein intake is not going to change; if anything its already high level may go even higher. One really has to change the total diet. Anything less than that is a cruel hoax on the population at large. It doesn't make sense."

The good news is that more profound dietary changes exert much more profound effects on health. Campbell found, for example, that diet appears to affect hormone function, which in turn, influences the age of puberty and other factors.

> *"One really has to change the total diet. Anything less than that is a cruel hoax on the population at large. It doesn't make sense."*
>
> **Dr. T. Colin Campbell**

"Menarche—a girl's first period—starts between fifteen and nineteen years of age in China, whereas it is twelve to thirteen in the United States," Campbell said. "As you know, a later age of menarche is correlated with a lower rate of breast cancer, at least when comparing different populations. So this later age of menarche in China is indicative of disease prevention in a sense."

What causes the difference in the age of puberty? The onset of puberty is triggered when a girl reaches a certain point in her growth. If she is on a high-fat, low-fiber diet that accelerates growth, she will have an early puberty and a higher risk of breast cancer later in life. "Of course, that is also the kind of diet that tends to elevate circulating estrogen levels," Campbell said. "So I think a lot of breast cancer could be accounted for by an overly rapid early growth rate in the United States. Now, this doesn't mean that we can't bring breast cancer under control later in life. For women who grew fast in the beginning, the evidence suggests that, were they to change their diets later on in life, they should be able to set back the inevitable progression to breast cancer."

The Chinese have a different experience at the beginning of their reproductive years. They also have a very different experience at menopause, as Campbell points out. "Chinese physicians who have worked with me say there are less problems at that age than there appear to be in the West. One hypothesis, if this is true, is that, in the case of Western women where the estrogen levels are sustained at fairly high levels throughout their reproductive years because of their high-fat diets, when they reach menopause those estrogen levels drop precipitously to the natural baseline levels. For women on lower-fat diets, these circulating estrogen levels are somewhat lower during the reproductive years, so they don't drop so markedly at menopause. The more rapid drop that we see in Western women may put them at higher risk for the adverse effects associated with metabolic adjustment, such as with calcium loss, for example."

The benefits of lower-fat diets, then, are not just fewer problems with hot flashes and mood swings. There are also 80 percent fewer hip fractures in China, compared to Western countries.

Westerners can take advantage of the benefits of plant-based diets themselves. Adapting is much easier than many people might imagine, as Campbell found out in his own family. "We started changing our diet when our children came along, and we have been changing ever since. I really don't see that a change, if desired, is that big of a deal. In the short run, people who are accustomed to a high-salt, high-fat diet are not going to like healthier foods at first. But if they have a little patience, they will find that after two or three months, perhaps longer, they adapt to new tastes. And then they discover new tastes that they never realized were there before."

From Prevention to Treatment

Asian traditions have contributed to our knowledge of how dietary changes help prevent illness. They have also provided novel treatments. One of the best known examples comes from Anthony Sattilaro, M.D., who was the President of Methodist Hospital in Philadelphia. In 1978, Dr. Sattilaro was diagnosed with prostate cancer. In older men, prostate cancer often follows a very slow course. But in younger men, like Dr. Sattilaro, prostate cancer is a grave disease. Modern medicine has done little to change the prognosis. When Dr. Sattilaro was found to have prostate cancer that had spread throughout his body, he was told to prepare for his death.

I met Dr. Sattilaro almost 10 years later, in 1986. Not only was he alive; he was youthful and vigorous. His cancer was gone, so far as his doctors could tell, and foods seemed to have played a major role in the change. And, a bit later on, other foods may have played a very malignant role. But first, the beginning of the story.

"I became the President of Methodist Hospital in 1977," Sattilaro said. "In May of 1978, in between all kinds of meetings with planners and builders, I went for my annual physical. A chest X-ray was routine at that time. About an hour after I got back to my office, I got a call from radiology.

"The radiologist said, 'How do you feel?' I said, 'I feel well. I'm too busy to be sick.' He said, 'You've got something in your left lung.' So I walked to the second floor to the radiology department, and sure enough, there was a golf-ball-sized lesion in the left lung. He thought it was in the lung, but said it might be in the rib. We then did a bone scan, which showed lesions in three areas of the skull, the right shoulder, two vertebrae, the entire sternum, and the left sixth rib.

"This was *not* in the program for the day. It wasn't on the calendar. It was such a crashing experience, realizing that your whole world was coming to an end. Cancer, to me, was a death sentence. Nothing was in perspective anymore. The biopsy results showed prostate cancer with metastases."

The cancer had begun in the prostate, but had metastasized, that is spread, to his bones. The result is often severe pain as the cancer grows within the bone.

"Cancer of the prostate in patients under 50 is a terminal disease. There are no survivors. After 50, the disease is very different. I had seen any number of patients who were 75 or 80 who had cancers of the prostate which were relatively benign.

"I knew the surgeon very well, and I also happened to be going to an internist who, by chance, was an oncologist and a good friend. I was told, literally, to get my affairs in order. I wasn't prepared to do that. I had just turned 48. The question was, why me? This is wrong. I went through that kind of agonizing, without much spiritual support, nothing to hold onto, and with all of the scientific data saying you're going to die and you have to get ready to do that. And I did. I put all of my affairs in order.

"I went back to work quickly. Work was a placebo for the pain. But I was then taking large doses of narcotics, and they finally put me on a thing called Brompton's mixture, which is morphine, cocaine, and Compazine. It's used in hospices. The morphine gave you a euphoria, but made you very nauseated, so the Compazine cut the vomiting down. The cocaine gave you an 'up' for the 'down' you get after the morphine. With the help of my assistant, I was able to block out interviews. I would wait until my speech wasn't slurred, and I'd be able to look as though I was operating pretty well.

"Then my father died with terminal cancer throughout his body. He died at Methodist Hospital. We went to the burial plot in central New Jersey, right near the little town where I had grown up. My mother was there, and we buried him on the seventh of August.

"Afterward, I got on the New Jersey Turnpike. It was beastly hot. There were two hitchhikers, and I picked them up. One fell asleep in the back seat. The other one was named Sean McLean, and we got to talking. I told him about the sad event I had just experienced, my father's death, and that I was dying, that I was going to be dead in a year or so. And he said very glibly to me, which annoyed the hell out of me, 'You don't have to die, Doc, cancer's easy to cure.'

"First of all, that's a very adolescent response to this great doctor, who knows that cancer isn't easy to cure. Here was somebody, a guy who was a cook, certainly not in my educational class, saying by absolute faith that it was easy to cure. And I have to say that I just dismissed him. He had graduated from cooking school, and he and his friend were going to South Carolina for a holiday before going to work. But something made him hook on to me. He said, 'We'll get off with you in Philadelphia. We're going to take you to a natural foods store.' Well, that was the last thing I was interested in. I have never had any real interest in food, and to this day I don't, except from what's happened to me. Meals were always very quick.

"So we went to the natural foods store, and I was utterly repelled by it. I thought natural foods were for people who just couldn't afford to eat meat and that they were all strange people who were against the Vietnam war and so on. I had the wildest ideas about vegetarians and people who ate natural foods.

"I went back to the hospital and I proceeded to do my work. Then about two weeks later I got a whole packet of information from these guys, with 67 cents postage due. It was about macrobiotics. Well, I looked at it and it was just pure garbage to me. The whole series of anecdotal stories saying 'I ate this way, and I did A, B, C, D, E and I got well.' You and I have seen that for any kind of thing. Vitamin C does it, or my trip with yoga does it, or all sorts of things. But something caught my eye. There was a physician who gave a testimonial. It was articulately done, and she was living in Philadelphia. So, I said, what the hell. It's my dime. I'll just call her.

"I remember the night very clearly. Her husband answered. I told him who I was, and I said, 'Tell me about your wife. She claims that she's had some really good results with this macrobiotic stuff.' And he said, 'Oh Doc, she's marvelous when she eats that way, but she hates the food. And she's now dying of cancer in the hospital. She can't eat that way.'

"She had abandoned the diet. I got intrigued by his very firm belief that diet was instrumental in her breast cancer. Here was a hormonally sensitive tumor of the breast, and I had prostate cancer, which is also hormone-related. And for whatever reasons, I guess it was a combination of pain, desperation, desolation, and just not wanting to die, I then decided that I would pursue the macrobiotic thing.

"I looked up the macrobiotic people in Philadelphia. And that was a vision to behold. I went to their house. I had to take my shoes off. And I sat down in the study of this very Asian-looking house on the outskirts of Philadelphia. This young fellow looked at my face, and looked at my eyes, and diagnosed my cancer using Asian methods, which I have learned since. He said, 'We can get you well.' And he wanted me to start on this very rigid diet, and I said, 'Well, I can't, I'm going to Italy next week.' He said, 'I beg you not to leave the United States. This is very important. You must get on this diet.' Well, I said okay.

> *"Then I started taking it [macrobiotics] seriously for a couple of reasons. Three weeks after I started the diet, I was able to throw all of the drugs away."*
>
> **Dr. Anthony Sattilaro**

"His wife gave me a cooking lesson on Saturday. I went out to buy this stuff, and it was just a complete blunder. First of all, I'd never been in the kitchen. I come from an Italian family where men never went into the kitchen. So I didn't know how to turn the stove on. To this day, I'm still clumsy in the kitchen. And I blew up the pot of brown rice. It was just a mess. An absolute mess. And I sat down and cried.

"So, I talked to them, and they were really nice. They said 'Well, why don't you come and eat with us? You can take your lunch to the hospital.' Well, I didn't know what I was getting into. It was a real community, a commune. The first night I went there, it seemed very strange, sitting on the floor and eating with chopsticks.

"But it was a challenge to me, because as I sat and listened to his lectures, everything that he was talking about was completely the opposite of what I had been taught. He taught me the five-element theory of diagnosis, how we interplay with nature, and the unified theory of disease. None of those things had ever been part of my medical training. We talked about problems with lungs, problems with kidneys, and so forth. They believe that there is an intermingling of all of these systems. It took me a long time to come to grips with that and then start realizing that it worked. Nobody at the hospital minded much, because I wasn't doing anything but bringing my food in. People were mostly sympathetic. They said, well, he's dying. What the hell. We'll kind of support somebody who's dying.

"Then I started taking it seriously for a couple of reasons. Three weeks after I started the diet, I was able to throw all of the drugs away. I didn't have to take any more morphine. The pain disappeared. When you have chronic pain, to get a day free, you'd have conversations with the devil. That's how debilitating pain is.

> *"Here was a case of a person who had had documented cancer, who had some things go radically differently in his life. The cancer was gone."*
>
> **Dr. Anthony Sattilaro**

"Well, that was the first step. I stayed in the community, although the people there were entirely different from me. They were 25 years younger than I was, with a whole set of values that was totally different, living very simple lives, eating food that had virtually no taste to it, forcing me to chew everything a hundred times. I could not say that I enjoyed the food at all, but I couldn't argue with the fact that I was feeling better.

By winter, when I was supposed to be going downhill, my hemoglobin levels were going up. I was feeling better; I had increased energy. By Easter time, I was back to my old self. And nobody could believe it.

"Then September came, and I had my annual X-ray. We took the X-ray, and that made history. Here was a case of a person who had had documented cancer, who had some things go radically differently in his life. The cancer was gone.

"Well, that was enough for me to start dealing with my cynicism. I still could not accept the society that I had been drawn into, because it was totally foreign to me. But I had to give credence to the fact that maybe there was something here.

"Things were going well at the hospital. It was building and growing. People were excited that I was well, although not very excited that I was eating a loony kind of diet and bringing chopsticks in, but I did it all with a sense of humor. That was the time when it was brought out that humor has an effect on disease. I treated it all as a big game. I just made up my mind that I would get well and went along with the whole show.

"So, in my private life I became a classical macrobiotic doing everything, including sleeping on a futon, having a gas stove in my apartment, and never wearing any synthetic clothes; everything was cotton. It was a 180-degree switch. Then I met Jean Kohler, who was a musicologist who had had pancreatic cancer. He wrote *Healing Miracles Through Macrobiotics*. I read that book, and I was inspired by talking to him and to his wife on the phone. His cancer had disappeared, and he attributed it to the diet. So I stayed on it and got very involved with the macrobiotic community. And the more I read, the more I became seduced by the whole concept that everything was upside down in the West, that we were starting from the wrong side."

> *"The remarkable thing about all of this was that I started getting better. By winter, when I was supposed to be going downhill, my hemoglobin levels were going up. And nobody could believe it."*
>
> **Dr. Anthony Sattilaro**

Sattilaro looked and felt terrific. He began to write of his experiences and to give lectures to audiences seeking the same cure he had apparently found. He felt so good, in fact, that he was tempted to believe he no longer needed the diet he was on. "I had thought about quitting," he said, "simply because I was now well. And what the hell, why did I need to do it any more? But they made it very clear that the cancer would come back and warned me that if it should come back, it would be very hard to cure it a second time. So I was terrified and, at the same time, seduced by the whole thing.

"It's eight years now. Why hasn't the cancer come back? They never took the cancer out. The cancer's still in the prostate. They don't feel it. Why did it go into remission? Where is it?

"It's fine for oncologists to say this is an unexplained remission. I think it's more responsible to explain the remission. We can't just simply laugh it off. After all, if I am a case that did get well with all these variables, why not use those variables in a lot of people? It would be terrific to test it. There are enough data now to show that certain types of cancer occur with less frequency among vegetarians. Seventh-day Adventists are a classic example of that. People who live in Asia are classic examples of that. And now we're able to collect pretty good data from Asia. I think it would be good to test it. Certainly for prevention. As a cure? I used it as a cure. Whether it cured me or not, I have no idea."

In spite of his experiences, Dr. Sattilaro never rejected Western medicine. As a physician trained in diagnosis and treatment, and as an administrator of a major metropolitan hospital which had helped a great many people, he saw the value of the Western medical tradition. Eastern medicine should be added to it, not used to simply replace it. "No way. We have Western minds. We have a system of thinking called logic that's got an Aristotelian base. But we also can't dismiss all of that knowledge of the East. The East is a complement to what we have in the West.

"The first step, obviously, is to get rid of the high-fat diet and go to high-fiber. Ten years ago, this was considered a radical idea. Now look at the television commercials with all the cereals competing. Of course, that's not the answer. It's a step. It's certainly better than ham and eggs."

A macrobiotic diet is a dramatic shift from a standard American diet. Its foods come from Asian culinary traditions, and explanations of its effect are derived from ancient Chinese medical concepts. So Western doctors and laypersons alike need a bit of effort to come to grips with it.

"When I went into macrobiotics, I didn't do it because I wanted to," Sattilaro said. "I had no choice. I don't think that an American public that doesn't know it's ill, and particularly a physician public that doesn't know how food affects the body, is anywhere near ready to make that kind of a leap. It takes a lot of energy and effort, because it is a life-style change, and I don't think most Americans want a life-style change. We are now addicted to the method, 'Doctor, get me well.' And doctor does get somebody well in many diseases."

Perhaps that is part of the reason Dr. Sattilaro finally did drop the diet. In spite of his own acknowledgment that abandoning the diet might cause the return of the cancer, he took that risk. "In the last three years, I haven't done macrobiotics. I went off the diet deliberately three years ago, to test the hypothesis that vegetarianism alone would still sustain me. I slowly went to a balanced vegetarian diet that included fish. Then I added chicken to the diet. I had three years of nonmacrobiotics to compare with five years of macrobiotics. And there was no cancer."

However, emerging health problems made him return to the macrobiotic diet, after his three-year experiment with more permissive diets.

"I've gone back," he said. "That experiment's over, because of the edema, the swelling, that I have in my hands. I'm going to try the macrobiotic approach to get my whole system back in balance."

But he did not get back in balance. As he had previously predicted, his cancer returned. In July, 1989, I spoke to him for the last time. He had resumed the use of pain-killers, which at times caused him to become quite groggy. He knew that the end was near.

Dr. Sattilaro was never sure that the regimen he followed could take credit for his decade-long reprieve from cancer. Nor do we know whether, had he not deviated from the diet, first to fish, then to chicken, he would have been able to keep his cancer at bay.

But it is clear that humble foods from the plant kingdom have enormous power, both to prevent disease and to alter its course—power that we have barely begun to tap. There are many variations on healthful diets, from diets based mainly on raw foods, to macrobiotic menus drawn from traditional Asian cuisine, to diets including the full range of vegetarian foods.

It is my hope that the wealth of knowledge and experience presented by the experts in this volume will illuminate much of what is already known about the power of foods and will intrigue the reader to explore those areas which are only beginning to be understood.

References

Chapter 1

1. Castelli WP. Epidemiology of Coronary Heart Disease, *Am J Medicine* 1984:76(2A):4-12.

Chapter 3

1 Moertel CG. On Lymphokines, Cytokines, and Breakthroughs. *JAMA* 1986;256:3141.

2. National Research Council. 1982. *Diet, Nutrition, and Cancer.* Washington: National Academy Press.

3. Armstrong B, Doll R. Environmental factors and cancer incidence and mortality in different countries, with special reference to dietary practices. *Int J Cancer* 1975;15:617-31.

4. Hirayama T. Epidemiology of breast cancer with special reference to the role of diet. *Prev Med* 1978; 7:173-195.

5. Rose DP, et al. Effect of a low-fat diet on hormone levels in women with cystic breast disease. 1. Serum steroids and gonadotropins. *JNCI* 1987;78(4):6233-26.

6. Ingram DM, et al. Effect of low-fat diet on female sex hormone levels. *JNCI* 1987;79(6):1225-29.

7. Kagawa Y. Impact of Westernization on the nutrition of Japanese: changes in physique, cancer, longevity and centenarians. *Prev Med* 1978;7:205-17.

Chapter 4

1. U.S. Department of Agriculture Food Safety and Inspection Service. *Nationwide beef microbiological baseline data collection program: steers and heifers,* October 1992-September 1993. Washinton, D.C.: U.S. Department of Agriculture, 1994.

2. Hergenrather J, et al. Pollutants in breast milk of vegetarians. *New Eng J Med* 1981;304:792

Chapter 5

1. Brand JC, et al. Plasma glucose and insulin responses to traditional Pima Indian meals. *Am J Clin Nutr* 1990;51:416-20.

2. Barnard RJ, et al. Response of non-insulin-dependent diabetic patients to an intensive program of diet and exercise. *Diabetes Care* 1982;5(4):370-74.

3. Barnard RJ, et al. Long-term use of a high-complex-carbohydrate, high-fiber, low-fat diet and exercise in the treatment of NIDDM patients. *Diabetes Care* 1983;6(3):268-73.

4. Scott FW. Cow milk and insulin-dependent diabetes mellitus: is there a relationship? *Am J Clin Nutr* 1990:51:489-91.

5. Karjalainen J, Martin JM, Knip M, et al. A bovine albumin peptide as a possible trigger of insulin-dependent diabetes mellitus. *N Engl J Med* 1992;327:302-7.

6. Kolata G. How important is dietary calcium in preventing osteoporosis? *Science* 1986;233:519-20.

7. Zemel MB. Role of the sulfur-containing amino acids in protein-induced hypercalciuria in men. *J Nutr* 1981; 111:545.

8. Hegsted M, et al. Urinary calcium and calcium balance in young men as affected by level of protein and phosphorus intake. *J Nutr* 1981;111:553.

9. Mazess R. Bone mineral content of North Alaskan Eskimos. *Am J Clin Nutr* 1974;27:916-25.

10. Simoons FJ. A geographic approach to senile cataracts: possible links with milk consumption, lactase activity, and galactose metabolism. *Digestive Diseases and Sciences* 1982;27(3):257-64.

11. Virag R, Bouilly P, Frydman D. Is impotence an arterial disorder? A study of arterial risk factors in 440 impotent men. *Lancet* 1985;1:181-84.

Chapter 6

1. Wurtman RJ. Aspartame: possible effect on seizure susceptibility. *Lancet* 1985;2:1060.

2. Camfield PR, Camfield CS, Dooley JM, Gordon K, Jollymore S, Weaver DF. Aspartame exacerbates EEG spike-wave discharge in children with generalized absence epilepsy: a double-blind controlled study. *Neurology* 1992; 42: 1000-03.

3. Janssen PJCM, van der Heijden CA. Aspartame: review of recent experimental and observational data. *Toxicology* 1988;50: 1-26

4. Yokogushi H, Wurtman RJ. Meal composition and plasma amino acid ratios: effect of various proteins on carbohydrates, and of various protein concentrations. *Metabolism* 1986;35(9):837-842.

5. Seltzer S, et al. The effects of dietary tryptophan on chronic maxillofacial pain and experimental pain tolerance. *J Psychiatric Res* 1983;17:181-86.

6. Seltzer S, et al. Alteration of human pain thresholds by nutritional manipulation and L-tryptophan supplementation. *Pain* 1982; 13:385-93.